The Life-Transforming
Diet

The Life-Transforming Diet

New Meal Choices
Updated Edition
ADDED NUTRITION & FITNESS GUIDELINES

Based on

Health and Psychological Principles of Maimonides

and other Classical Sources

David J. Zulberg

Supported and Expanded with the
Latest Health and Nutritional Principles

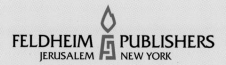

FELDHEIM PUBLISHERS
JERUSALEM   NEW YORK

ISBN 978-1-59826-977-2

First published 2007
Corrected edition, 2009
New, updated edition, 2014

FELDHEIM PUBLISHERS
POB 43163/ Jerusalem, Israel

208 Airport Executive Park
Nanuet, NY 10954
www.feldheim.com

10   9   8   7   6   5   4   3   2   1

Book design: Michelle Levy, Jerusalem Typesetting
Typesetting and layout: Raphaël Freeman, Jerusalem Typesetting

Printed in Israel

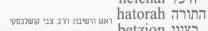

יום ד' כ"ו שבט התשס"ז

בס"ד

מכתב ברכה

הרמב"ם בספר ההלכות שלו – ספר היד החזקה העוסק כולו בענייני המצוות וחיובי התורה, הכניס בו ג"כ את ענייני הרפואה, אשר לכאורה אינם אלא כמילי דעלמא ואינם שייכים כלל לספר הלכות. ומדוע הכניסם הרמב"ם בספר ההלכות.

אלא שהגמרא בשבת (פב.) מביאה, דרב הונא שאל את בנו רבה, מאי טעמא לא שכיחת קמיה דרב חסדא דמחדדן שמעתיה? אמר ליה, מאי איזיל לגביה דכי אזילנא לגביה מותיב לי במילי דעלמא, אמר לי מאן דעייל לבית הכסא לא ליתיב בהדיא ולא ליטרח טפי, דהאי כרכשתא אתלת שיני יתיב, דילמא משתמטא שיני דכרכשתא ואתי לידי סכנה. אמר ליה, הוא עסיק בחיי דברייתא ואת אמרת במילי דעלמא כל שכן זיל לגביה. ע"כ.

כלומר, רבה בנו של רב הונא נמנע מללכת אל שיעוריו של רב חסדא בטענה, שעוסקים הם במילי דעלמא – ענייני רפואה. והוכיחו רב הונא על כך שטועה הוא בחשיבות לימוד חכמת הרפואה, ומחמת שיש בה "חיי דברייתא", היא נכללת בכלל דברי תורה, וכל שכן שיש חשיבות רבה ללמוד אצלו.

ומבואר שרב הונא אשר היה ראש ישיבה וכל מעייניו היה בלימוד התורה והרבצתה, בכל זאת ראה חשיבות גדולה בענייני תורת הרפואה ואף הקדימה לענייני התורה.

וכדברינו כתב בפירושו הבונה לעין יעקב בשבת שם וז"ל: מילי דעלמא היה קורא רבה לכל דבר שאינו לימוד בתורה והודיעו אביו שחיי שחיי האדם ובריאותו הוא לימוד ראוי וצריך לכל בן תורה כדי שיוכל להנות בה, ואינו מילי דעלמא וכו'. ואמר לו שתיקון הגוף קודם לתיקון הנפש בזמן ובטבע. ע"כ.

ואולי יש לומר שעל זה סמך הרמב"ם שהכניס בספר ההלכות שלו את ענייני הרפואה, כדי לגלות על חשיבותם ומעלתם, ועל הצורך בידיעתם ולימודם חשוב כלימוד תורה. וכשידע כראוי עניינים אלו, יישנה את אורחות חייו והנהגותיו ויקיים כראוי את חיוב התורה של "וחי בהם."

ועל כן שמחתי לראות את חיבורו של האברך החשוב הרה"ג ר' דוד זולברג שליט"א, אשר בעמל ובגיעה רבה ליקט בירר וערך בצורה מסודרת ויפה, כדי להקל על הלומד להבין לאשורם את דבריו של הרופא הגדול הרמב"ם, ולנהוג על פיהם.

ואין לי אלא לברכו יהא רעוא שיתקבל חיבורו זה בעלמא ויזכה להגדיל תורה ולהאדירה להוציא עוד ספרים כהנה כידו הטובה עליו, ברחבות הדעת ושלות הנפש.

בברכת התורה

שמואל קמנצקי
Rabbi S. Kamenetsky

2018 Upland Way
Philadelphia, Pa 19131

Home: 215-473-2798
Study: 215-473-1212

בס"ד ג' כ' תולדות תשס"ו

לכבוד ר' זאב שליט"א נ"י

קבלתי מכ' דרישת דרולא לבן/בת ציון

מורשי את הדברים.

דרך שלום ולא ירו בין כך לכרמלא של כל

כראל, לברוך רפ"ח חיים וקיימים ישרים ונאמרים.

בברכת אל פון ירושמם כתוב כן ונודע ישראל

ידיד לעולמים

הכותב דברי השלום

[חתימה]

Rabbi Dovid Zulberg has made a valuable contribution by the publication of his masterful work "The Rambam's Life Transforming Diet". The Rambam's assertion that diet and exercise are the key to good health is well known. So too is his personal guarantee that whoever follows his system will live a full and healthy life, one of the most amazing statements in all of Rabbinic literature. Yet despite that there are few takers and little interest. It is perhaps the Rambam's penchant for brevity and terseness that set his clear and unequivocal language beyond the pale of everyone but the intellectual elite. Rabbi Zulberg has adorned the Rambam's principles with a presentation which makes these essentials accessible to the masses. For this alone he deserves our accolades.

There is a second issue which is of equal importance and deserves mention. Having achieved the limits of bounty and availability of all foods at all times and in all localities, our American culture has succeeded in making an art and a preferred life style out of indulgence. Restraint has very little appeal where linguistics have elevated gourmandry to the titular heights of cuisine, culinary art and gourmet living. Limits are for those of limited means if they exist at all. Rabbi Zulberg has done an important service in providing a popular setting and scintillating attractiveness for what is usually resisted for its restrictiveness and deprivation. He has endowed regulated behavior with an aura of fun and excitement. If, Hashem willing, he will succeed in having brought the Rambam's living system to the attention of the people and precipitate an active interest in its diet and principles of moderation and activity, his contribution would be considered monumental. May he enjoy success in this and in all his endeavors,

27th Teves 5767

Rabbi Yisroel Haleivi Belsky

Abraham J. Twerski, M.D.
Gateway Rehabilitation Center
Moffett Run Road
Aliquippa, Pennsylvania 15001

Maimonides (Rambam) is considered one of the greatest physicians of antiquity. His greatness is primarily of historic value, because in the 12th century, he had no access to the miracles of modern medicine. He had no antibiotics, no cortisone, no x-ray, and no surgical anesthesia. However, there is one area where his opinion may be authoritative even today, and that is nutrition. There are so many different theories today about what constitutes proper nutrition, that modern science cannot claim superiority in this area.

Maimonides was court physician to the Sultan of Egypt. The Sultan once asked him, "How can I tell that you are a competent physician? You have never treated me for any illness, because I am healthy." Maimonides responded, "The reason you have not been ill is because you have followed my instructions. The skill of a physician is to prevent one from becoming ill." Maimonides describes a course for healthy living, and makes the bold claim that whoever adheres to his instructions will not become ill, and will die only of old age.

The halachic works of Maimonides are authentic Torah. Maimonides' chapter on nutrition is in his halachic works; hence it has the status of Torah. Our great Torah scholars were very cautious with their words. A statement by Maimonides guaranteeing good health if one adheres to his regimen has the force of halachah.

David Zulberg has taken Maimonides' instructions for proper nutrition, accompanied by other suggestions for proper living, and made them available in an easily understood form. It is a major contribution to a field where there is so much controversy and confusion. As a codifier of Jewish law, Maimonides' opinion has great impact even today. Zulberg's work may prove that this is equally true of his instructions on nutrition.

Abraham J. Twerski, M.D.
Founder & Medical Director Emeritus

Rabbi Dovid Goldwasser
Khal Bais Yitzchok
Brooklyn, NY 11223

הרב דוד גאלדוואסער
רב דקהל בית יצחק
ברוקלין, ניו יורק

בס"ד

Tzom Gedalyah 5766

In today's times much attention is being focused on issues of diet and weight loss. Because of its popularity, many have become self-styled experts in how to maintain the "perfect" body weight. However, this area of life, too, requires *daas Torah*.

A few decades ago R' Moshe Feinstein *zt'l* was asked a *sheiloh* concerning dieting. R' Moshe draws a significant line of demarcation between normative dieting, and crash dieting which he did not permit. From this most important *teshuvah*, many have come to the understanding that matters of health and diet have to be addressed from a Torah perspective, as we learn in *Tehillim (119:105)* "נר לרגלי דבריך ואור לנתיבתי" -- Your word is a lamp for my feet and a light for my path."

Having had the privilege, for the past decade, of working with people suffering from eating disorders, it is a particular *simcha* for me to see that Rav Dovid Zulberg has put out a monumental work entitled *The Life-Transforming Diet*. Now thousands of our brethren who wish to know the Torah's outlook on dieting and good health will have a clear and authoritative work that is well-organized and user friendly.

Rav Zulberg bases his work upon the principles set forth by the *Rambam*. The *Rambam* writes *(Hilchos Dei'os, Chapter 4, Halacha 15)*, "Most illnesses come to a person because he eats foods that are bad for him, or because he fills his stomach and eats excessively – *achilah gasoh*."

In *Mishlei* (21:32) the *posuk* tells us שמר פיו ולשונו שמר מצרות נפשו – one who guards his mouth and his tongue guards his soul from troubles" This has been interpreted to mean that if a person will guard his mouth from eating foods that are harmful or from overeating he will guard his soul from troubles.

I am confident that this book will be well received and will replace secular books of this genre. All who read it are מקיים the *mitzvah* "ונשמרתם מאד לנפשתיכם -- You shall greatly beware for your souls" *(Devorim 4:15)*.

I wish the author *hatzlacha rabbah* in this endeavor and in all areas of life. May he be *zoche* to be counted among the "*matzdikei harabbim shetzidkosom omedes lo'ad.*"

Hametzapeh l'yeshuah
Rabbi Dovid Goldwasser

LAWRENCE KELEMEN
P.O. Box 34490
JERUSALEM ▲ 91342 ▲ ISRAEL

בס"ד
לייב קעלעמען
ת.ד. 34490
ירושלים 91342

"The intellect is the rebbe and the guide that a person receives from the Creator to guard, advise and educate him all the days of his life."

So Rav Yerucham Levovitz *ztz"l* taught his students in a 1935 *shmuess* to the students of the Mir Yeshiva in Poland (*Daas Chochmo Umussar* v. 1, p. 11). The Mirrer Moshgiach stressed that we are halachicly bound to live intelligent lives, and that acting foolishly constitutes a real transgression (ibid., p. 24). His words obligate us to carefully consider whether our conduct conforms to the dictates of what he calls *derech eretz* - reason applied to reality. Rav Yerucham helps us understand why our greatest *rishonim* and *achronim* took time out of their busy schedules to study principles of health and fitness, and why they included recommendations about diet, exercise and sleep in their Torah discourses.

During centuries of exile from our land, foreign perspectives penetrated pockets within the Jewish community. Among these was a belief that G-d cares only about ritual observance, but not about *derech eretz*. Even today, amidst a virtual renaissance of Jewish learning, there remain some Jews who are unfamiliar with our responsibility to live intelligently and protect our health. This ignorance has had grave consequences in many cases.

R' David Zulberg has performed an invaluable service by assembling a plan for healthy living that is consistent both with the advice of our sages and the findings of modern medicine. His work is unique among diet/exercise guides in its reasonable tone and moderate approach. It is not only enjoyable, but will earn the respect of Torah scholars and medical professionals alike.

Historically, partial observance of the Torah eroded respect for our tradition. Full observance of both the letter and spirit of our tradition produced admiration of Torah both within and outside the observant community. May David Zulberg's book be a source of *kiddush Hashem* in our generation.

בידידות
א"ג
לייב קעלעמען

DR. CHARLENE WOLBERG

MBBCh (Wits)
Pr. No. 1582232
LINKSFIELD NUTRITION MED-CLINIC

SUITE 200, MEDICAL CENTRE
LINKSFIELD PARK CLINIC
24 - 12TH AVENUE, ORANGE GROVE
LINKSFIELD WEST, JHB
TEL.: +27 11 640-7763/4

E-MAIL: scwolberg@telkomsa.net

⌂ P. O. BOX 29178
SANDRINGHAM
2131
SOUTH AFRICA
FAX: +27 11 640-7765

12th December 2006

Obesity (from the Latin obesus, one who has become plump from eating) first appears in western medical literature in Thomas Venner's Via Recta in 1620. However, many centuries before, Rambam had already addressed this. A disease which has been reported almost 400 years ago in the western medical literature, but who's incidence continues to rise in epidemic proportions.

Obesity is a chronic multifaceted disease that requires multimodal management. To archive success significant life changes need to be made. Dietary manipulation, increase in physical activity and behaviour modification need to be introduced. The shortcoming of many diet programmes is that they focus on only one aspect of the problem, without acknowledging obesity has multiple causes. A holistic balanced approach is required if one hopes to achieve and maintain success in weight management.

THE LIFE TRANSFORMING DIET has presented a programme based on Maimonides' teachings on health. It puts forward a weight loss programme that addresses dietary, exercise and behavioural aspects of eating.

One of the misconceptions people have about weight loss is that rapid and large changes are desirable or even possible. The importance of gradual and sustained changes is emphasized in this book.

Our medical teachers often remind us that teachings which were once regarded as outdated and obsolete regularly come back into practice when new facts about them are discovered.

The understanding of proper nutrition is returning to the principles espoused by the Rambam.

It is my belief that this book will be of great benefit to those that read it and apply its principles appropriately.

Charlene Wolberg

Charlene Wolberg MD, Medical Director

ACKNOWLEDGMENTS

I would like to thank the ultimate Healer for allowing me to reach this stage. Writing this book has been a wonderful, multi-faceted adventure.

I am grateful to my Rashei HaYeshivos, HaGaon HaRav Zvi Kushelevsky, *shlita*, and HaGaon HaRav Binyomin Moskowitz, *shlita*, for the productive years that I spent learning in their *yeshivos*. It is there that I gained the tools to be able to research and write this book. I was also instilled with an excitement for learning all of Rambam's works and their commentaries.

A special thank you to R' Yaakov and Mendy Feldheim for their enthusiasm and confidence in this book. I am also grateful to the whole Feldheim team including Rabbi David Kahn and the editorial, design and production staff. I especially appreciate my talented editor, Mrs. Deena Nataf, for her excellent editing, sharp insights and patience.

I would also like to thank the following people who made valuable editorial contributions prior to the publishing stage: Dr. Charlene Wolberg for her time and expert nutritional advice. Allan Zulberg, Rabbi and Mrs. Yosef Leib Rakov, Dr. Lisa Aiken and Dr. Fred Rosner for their constructive comments. Finally, my mother, Linda Zulberg, who devoted her time and capabilities the way only a dedicated mother can, at all hours of the night and through the many different versions of this book. She is a shining light, a true inspiration and a living example of the Life-Transforming Diet system.

I am indebted to the Gedolim, Rashei HaYeshivos and Rabbanim who gave me of their valuable time: HaGaon HaRav Zvi Kushelevsky, *shlita*, HaGaon HaRav Shmuel Kamenetsky, *shlita*, HaGaon HaRav Yisroel Belsky, *shlita*, Rabbi Dr. Abraham Twerski and Rabbi Lawrence Kelemen, for their constant excellent advice and support. Rabbi Dovid Goldwasser for his confidence and excitement in this project. My Rav, Rabbi Moshe Brown, Rabbi Peretz Steinberg, Rabbi Berel Wein and Rabbi Akiva Tatz.

Regarding Rambam's great works that were originally written in Arabic, I benefited from the following translations: *Medical works*: An English translation by E. Faris, H.E. Hoff, and A. Bar Sela called *Moses Maimonides: Two Treatises on the Regimen of Health* (Philadelphia: American Philosophical Society, 1964), another English translation by Gerrit Bos, first edition (Provo, Utah: Brigham Young University Press, 2002), a complete English translation of all Rambam's medical works by Dr. Fred Rosner (Haifa: Maimonides Research Institute, 1984–1994) and a complete Hebrew translation of all Rambam's medical works by Dr. S. Munter (Jerusalem: Mosad HaRav Kook, 1957). *Moreh Nevuchim*: English translations include Shlomo Pines (Chicago: University of Chicago Press, 1963) and M. Friedlander (New York: Hebrew Publishing Co., 1881). Hebrew translations include Rabbi Yosef Kapach (Jerusalem: Mosad HaRav Kook, 1977). Each one of these translations was used extensively in the Rambam quotations throughout this book.

The Life-Transforming
Diet

CONTENTS

INTRODUCTION
THE LIFE-TRANSFORMING DIET DIFFERENCE

RAMBAM'S GUARANTEE

Imagine for a moment a world where almost every disease can be prevented and most people enjoy long and healthy lives. If we were able to visit this idyllic world we would probably try to absorb whatever we could of their lifestyle habits in order to emulate their successes in our own lives.

Unfortunately, we live in a very different world with frightening health statistics. More than half of the United States population is overweight or obese,[1] and many suffer from resultant health complications! Eating disorders abound, and we are flooded with conflicting advice and false promises to attain our dream of health. Confusion seems to be the norm. Ours is a world in which optimum health levels seem to be out of reach!

One of the greatest Jewish scholars in history tackled these issues. He gives us the means to make this dream a reality. I am referring to Rambam.[2]

In no uncertain terms, and without the slightest hesitation, Rambam writes the following mind-boggling guarantee to someone who follows his main principles of nutrition:

---

1. For these and other statistics, see the relevant Internet reference in Appendix E (page 323).
2. Rambam is an acronym for **R**abbeinu **M**oshe **b**en **M**aimon. He is known as Maimonides in Greek. Rambam lived from 1135 or 1138 to 1204. See Appendix B (page 305) for a more detailed discussion on his life.

> Whoever conducts himself in the ways we have set forth, I will *guarantee* that he will not get sick throughout his life.... He will not need a doctor and his body will be in perfect shape and remain healthy all his life.[3]

This assertion is found in Rambam's magnum opus, the *Mishneh Torah* – an authoritative halachic work which is an essential part of the Jewish tradition.

Indeed, this great Torah personality was also one of the foremost physicians in history. Authorities state that Rambam's advice about health and the prevention of disease remains relevant today. In the classical sources, *Migdal Oz* writes,[4] "Rambam's principles of health are clear, apply to all people, and everyone agrees with them." The *Kitzur Shulchan Aruch*[5] simply repeats many of Rambam's main nutritional principles almost verbatim. In our times, the well-known and -respected Rabbi Dr. Abraham J. Twerski, M.D., wrote to me, "I consider anything Rambam said about nutrition to be true. Furthermore, I consider Rambam's Guarantee to be ironclad." Similarly, Dr. Charlene Wolberg, a nutritionist and medical director of an obesity clinic, concludes that "The understanding of proper nutrition is returning to the principles espoused by the Rambam."[6]

3. *Mishneh Torah, Hilchos De'os* 4:20.
4. Commentary on *Hilchos De'os* 4:1 found in standard *Mishneh Torah* editions.
5. Chapter 32.
6. It is important to distinguish between ancient "medical remedies and prescriptions" and Rambam's health and nutrition advice. They are two completely different subjects. As the *Sefer Hakovetz* writes (*Hilchos De'os*, Chapter 4), "This is the very reason why Rambam left out all 'medical remedies and prescriptions' from his chapter on health and nutrition in *Mishneh Torah.*" (See also *Be'er Moshe* 6:159; *Sdei Chemed* 3–9, 5.)

In contrast, there seems to be a consensus that the "medical remedies and prescriptions" found in the Talmud should not be applied in our times. See Rav Sherira Gaon, *Otzar HaGeonim, Gittin* 68. Tosafos (*Mo'ed Katan* 11a) writes regarding the medical treatments found in the Talmud that they are not beneficial in our times. *Yam shel Shlomo* (*Chullin* 8:12) writes that it is actually forbidden to practice them. (See also Tosafos,

But "the proof of the pudding is in the eating" (no pun intended). A large part of the Yemenite Jewish population, which followed Rambam's main principles and teachings, had an average life span of one hundred years! This population lived in Yemen until about fifty years ago.

I can thankfully say that those who have taken on the principles of The Life-Transforming Diet have gained health, lost weight quickly and kept it off while experiencing a transformation of mind and body.

Rambam's amazing Guarantee is waiting to be realized by YOU.

It is possible to achieve longevity, outstanding health and a body which is in excellent shape. Let's put an end to the frightening health and weight-loss statistics! By reading this book, you are on your way to experiencing all the many rewards a healthy lifestyle promises.

ABOUT THIS BOOK

Health and Nutrition

The Life-Transforming Diet is based on time-tested principles, rooted in the teachings of Rambam, for gaining health and regulating weight – permanently! I specifically call them principles rather than rules because you will not feel restricted by them. Instead, you will be empowered to choose *how* to eat. The diet will give you the flexibility to create your own eating patterns in harmony with your personal lifestyle and preferences. Furthermore, principles are timeless and unchanging, whereas specific advice or theories may be disproved over time.

Avodah Zarah 24b; *Kesef Mishneh, Hilchos De'os* 4:18; Rema, *Even HaEzer* 156:3; *Shevet HaLevi*, vol. 3, 141:3; *Bris Olam* 477; *Chavas Yair* 234.)

The U.S. Dietary Guidelines, which by law (Public Law 101-445, Title III, 7 U.S.C. 5301 et seq.) are reviewed and updated if necessary, are published every five years. The process to create the Dietary Guidelines is a joint effort of the U.S. Department of Health and Human Services (HHS) and the U.S. Department of Agriculture (USDA). The Life-Transforming Diet empowers you to customize your own personal program and still fulfill current scientific fitness and nutritional requirements.

Rambam begins his famous chapter on health with the following advice:

> A person should eat only when he is hungry and he should drink only when he is thirsty.[7]

This sounds simple: We should listen to our bodies! However, we all know how hard this can be in practice. Our bodies have become used to bad habits and consequently can no longer be relied upon to accurately read the cues. Our goal is to reinstate the integrity of our natural internal systems. Then, we will eat when we are hungry and stop eating before satiation occurs – because that is what we do naturally.

Successful weight loss is not only about losing excess pounds. It's also about acquiring positive eating and lifestyle habits which are based on effective and timeless principles. Gradually we will relearn how to listen to and rely on our bodies. We will lose weight, but most important, maintaining our success will be a natural consequence of the positive habits developed during the process of losing weight and gaining health.

Habit Formation

Interestingly, Rambam places his advice on maintaining health in his *Hilchos De'os*, a section of *Mishneh Torah* which discusses emotional development

---

7. *Mishneh Torah, Hilchos De'os* 4:1.

and personal improvement! Elsewhere, Rambam writes explicitly that many of our bad food choices and bad eating habits originate from our learned perceptions.[8] It is clear that Rambam considered achieving optimum health as more than simply an issue of diet and exercise.

Most diets concentrate on the food itself with emphasis on outer results. After all, most people want to look better externally! The inner causative process is often ignored. But our external habits are the physical manifestations of inner motivational forces at work. Therefore, in order to achieve our aim of health and weight management, it is necessary to understand how our minds are involved in our eating habits. Then we will be able to create and cultivate positive eating and lifestyle habits and facilitate the achievement of our goals.

Practical Process

Sometimes we read or hear something inspirational, yet we fail to actually change as a result of this insight. What happened to that powerful moment of inspiration? I know people who have voluminous information on nutrition at their fingertips, but they're still trying to lose weight and gain health! Mere knowledge of nutritional and psychological principles is insufficient. We need to learn how to internalize our knowledge on a day-to-day basis. This is done through a precise plan of action, which will be implemented through the Phases of this program. Each Phase has been specifically designed from both a physical and a psychological perspective. The guidelines are absolutely clear and the principles are implemented at the right pace.

8. *Treatise on Asthma* 13:51.

A Gateway

If you need to lose weight, your body fat will melt away, transforming your outer appearance. You will feel and actually be much healthier and more energized. And you will even see an improvement in your emotional outlook.

For all these reasons, I have called my program The Life-Transforming Diet. This system of gaining health and losing weight will become a gateway to fulfilling your multi-faceted potential.

Before we continue, I have two requests:

First, please come with an open mind! This may sound obvious, but we all have our established opinions. Often, we are unaware that our perceptions actually limit our choices.[9] Why should we miss out on great opportunities – plus Rambam's Guarantee – just because we have become accustomed to certain opinions?

Second, I ask you to bear in mind that all the information in this book is interrelated, and it is impossible to form a clear picture of the Life-Transforming Diet until you have read the whole book.

Let me continue by telling you about what prompted me to change my life.

MY PERSONAL IMPETUS

As a teenager, I was healthy, fit and of normal weight. I always enjoyed snacking between meals. My favorites were chocolate, pastries, ice cream and potato chips. I always had an aversion to fruit, and I was a big fan of

---

9. In his *Moreh Nevuchim* (1:31), Rambam writes that a love for opinions to which we are habituated and with which we are reared can prevent us from seeing the truth.

burgers, fries and pizza. Yet I still remained in good shape because I was very active, and was satisfied by much smaller amounts of food.

This all took a sharp turn after I got married. The snacking continued between meals, but now I was also sitting down to large delicious meals every day, prepared by my talented wife. Very soon, I "needed" larger amounts of food and snacks to "satisfy" me. Additionally, I was studying for over twelve hours a day and exercise had become a word of the past. As you can imagine, by this point I was not exactly the fittest fiddle in town.

A few years later, I began experiencing severe heartburn. It was more than the normal discomfort to which I had become accustomed. This time my whole chest was on fire! I started popping antacids, but when nine a day didn't help, I decided it was time to visit a medical doctor.

The doctor took one look at me and diagnosed an ulcer. I was twenty-three years old at the time.

A few days later, a videoflouroscopy (camera down my throat) determined that I really had G.E.R.D. (gastro-esophageal reflux disorder). The doctor assured me that there was nothing to be concerned about. This was a very "normal" condition endured by millions worldwide. "A pill a day will keep the reflux away," he chuckled.

This "innocent" pill was an advanced antacid, but who cared? After all, it did the trick. My G.E.R.D. was "under control," and that was all that mattered.

At the same time, I would contract severe sinusitis at least four or five times a year. When it got really bad, I would return to my doctor. "Same thing again, eh?" he would say, writing a prescription for an antibiotic and a decongestant. Thus, I was used to an abundance of medications.

Still, I did not see myself as being so different from the average person. Mine were very common conditions. But my concerned, health-conscious mother made an appointment with a doctor of alternative medicine, and I went – to make her happy. I told the doctor about my state of health, and she insisted that my lifestyle would have to change. To be honest, I was not really convinced at the time, but I agreed to read the package insert of the medication I was taking for G.E.R.D.

The list of possible side effects was ferocious! I was a bit uncomfortable after reading it, as it included gastrointestinal disturbances, headache, taste disturbances, fatigue, and alterations in liver function test values. Also listed were cases of arthralgia, myalgia, peripheral edema, depression, hallucinations, confusion, vertigo, hematological changes, bruising, purpura, petechiae, jaundice, hepatitis, parasthesia, gynacomastia, impotence, hair thinning, photosensitivity, blurred vision, and interstitial nephritis sometimes resulting in renal failure… The list went on and on.

Yet all this was still insufficient to motivate me to change. I was happy with my eating habits and my lifestyle. But then people started making remarks about how I was putting on weight. I was also feeling very tired and lethargic a lot of the time, and the heartburn was persistently bad.

I had finally reached the point where I was prepared to entertain the possibility of making a change. I had to do something – but what?

My family doctor confirmed that many of my symptoms would certainly diminish if I lost the excess weight. But I didn't think I was that overweight; perhaps just a little "fuller" and "healthier" looking!

Little did I realize that I was at least thirty pounds overweight!

When I looked in the mirror, I saw what I wanted to see. Any external divergence from the perception of my "ideal self" was simply the mirror's distortion! Only after I had lost all the weight I needed to lose did this point finally hit home, when a friend remarked, "Wow, you look just like that picture on your mantelpiece." Only then did it dawn on me: he had met me a few years after the picture had been taken, but my perception of myself had never diverged from the image of that young and fit lad in the photograph. I had simply overlooked the evidence of the creeping pounds. Today, it is almost painful for me to look at pictures of myself at that heavy stage. I can hardly recognize myself.

It became clear to me that I had to improve my eating and lifestyle habits as well as lose weight. So we got some recipes from health-conscious family friends. To be honest, my new diet was fit for a horse! Everything on the menu was absolutely tasteless. It was Bland City, including greenish watery soup, brown, thick gooey rice and tasteless, rubbery burgers. Furthermore, the No list was a lot longer than the Yes list. I truly did respect my friends' advice, but I found it hard to contemplate eating this way even on a temporary basis. "Why not just have grass and mud?" I mumbled, dreading the possibility of never savoring tasty food again. "At least it'll be good for my complexion," I quipped.

So I started asking various "seasoned dieters" about weight loss. Sadly, those who claimed to be the greatest experts were overweight themselves! Though each one had lost weight at some stage, most of them had reverted back to their bad old habits, unable to maintain their weight losses.

The truth stared at me in the face: I could not find an option that worked for me. So I began to research the subject myself. I was astounded that there was very little on which the experts could agree. I had no desire to make difficult sacrifices when there was always another prominent professional with a different opinion! I was drowning in a sea of what felt like impractical, draconian rules. I didn't want to have to follow some sort of extreme program for the rest of my life.

Then I realized that the solution lay at the very root of our own tradition.

In ancient medicine, *prevention* of disease and nutrition played a central role, as Rambam writes:

> In the practice of medicine, the first and most important regimen is the one for the healthy, which insures that the existing state of health is not lost.[10]

> An expert physician who wants to guard his patient's health begins by improving [the latter's] diet.[11]

Rambam's works are filled with health and nutritional advice. Besides his well-known chapter on health,[12] he wrote ten major medical works, which include detailed discussions and explanations on health and nutrition.

Among Rambam's medical writings, I studied his *Regimen of Health, Treatise on Asthma, Medical Aphorisms, Causes of Symptoms, Treatise on Hemorrhoids, Galen's Art of Cure* and *Commentary on Hippocrates' Aphorisms*. I also found it necessary to study Rambam's other works on psychology and ethics. These include *Sefer HaMada,*[13] *Shemoneh Perakim,*[14] sections from *Moreh Nevuchim,*[15] *Introduction to Perek Chelek,*[16] *Letters*[17] and *Peirush HaMishnayos.*[18]

All Rambam's writings are interrelated. One sheds light on the other. They lay the foundation for understanding how the mind, the emotions and the body interact. Since Rambam's works are very concise and precise, anyone studying them needs many other scholarly explanations and commentaries in order to develop some of his main principles. As a result, I had the wonderful opportunity to delve into many additional classical writings.

---

10. *Regimen of Health* 2:1.
11. Introduction to *Peirush HaMishnayos.*
12. *Mishneh Torah, Hilchos De'os*, chapter 4.
13. The Book of Knowledge, which is the first volume of *Mishneh Torah.*
14. "Eight Chapters" (part of *Peirush HaMishnayos*) – Rambam's Introduction to *Pirkei Avos.*
15. Guide of the Perplexed.
16. *Perek Chelek* is the tenth chapter of tractate Sanhedrin.
17. *Iggeret Teiman*, etc.
18. Rambam's commentary on the Mishnah.

Thus, I began to research and write this book. It took me about five years to complete. Since I began following The Life-Transforming Diet, I have lost almost forty pounds! I have kept it off and never felt healthier. I can also thankfully say that others have experienced similar success.

We invite you, too, to join our Winners' Circle.

CHAPTER 1
RAMBAM'S RECIPE

According to ancient and medieval medicine, the health of the body is dependent not only on internal factors such as the body's strength and inner composition, but on six external factors as well. These six factors are called the *sex res non naturals*, or the "six non-naturals." In his *Treatise on Asthma*, Rambam discusses them:

> It is well-known that physicians have arranged the obligatory regimen of healthy and sick people into six essential categories:
>
> 1. Quality of surrounding air
>
> 2. Type of food and drink
>
> 3. Emotions
>
> 4. Exercise and rest
>
> 5. Sleeping and waking
>
> 6. Excretion and retention.

There is a seventh category of non-essential elements which affect the body only on occasion. They are bathing, massaging[1] and intimate relations.[2]

In his *Mishneh Torah*, Rambam further reduces the list into four fundamental principles of health (see below).

---

1. *Treatise on Asthma* 1:3.
2. Ibid., 1:4.

THE NUCLEUS

Rambam prescribes a recipe for achieving optimum health:

> The physicians have taught the following fundamental principle for health:
>
> A person who exercises and exerts himself greatly, does not satiate himself and has loose bowels,[3] will not become ill and his strength will increase, even if bad foods are eaten.
>
> But a person who does not exercise, delays relieving himself or suffers from constipation will suffer from pain all his life and his strength will fade, even if the correct foods are eaten and all the rules of medicine are kept.
>
> Overeating is like poison to the body and it is the main cause of all illness.
>
> Most illnesses are caused by unhealthy foods or by gorging oneself and overeating even healthy foods."[4]

In these few short lines, Rambam has listed the four main ingredients for achieving optimum health:

1. Food quantity

2. Exercise

3. Food quality

4. Waste management

---

3. I.e. tends to loose bowels, but certainly not to diarrhea.
4. *Mishneh Torah, Hilchos De'os* 4:14–15. Rambam continues: "King Solomon implied this in his wisdom: 'One who guards his mouth and his tongue guards himself from suffering' (*Mishlei* 21:23). He means to say, 'One who guards his mouth' from eating unhealthy food or overeating, 'and his tongue' from speaking only about his needs [guards himself from pain and suffering]."

However, Rambam seems to paint a different picture when he begins his most famous medical work, *Regimen of Health*:

> Hippocrates said, "The preservation of health lies in abstaining from satiation and avoiding exertion to the point of collapse." Contemplate how Hippocrates encompassed the general *regimen of health* in two principles, and they are:
>
> One should not satiate himself or over-exert himself, so that the benefits of movement and exercise are not lost.[5]

From this excerpt, it seems that our health depends on just two and not four main principles of health:

1. Food quantity
2. Exercise

There is no mention of food quality and waste management.

Primary Principles

Food Quantity

What would you say is better? Overeating the best quality foods or undereating poor quality foods?

I would have thought that the best quality food is always better than poor quality food! However, the opposite is true and this is the logic in Rambam's words:

> All physicians agree that eating a small quantity of bad foods is less harmful than overeating good and healthy foods. When a person eats bad foods without satiating oneself, the foods are digested well,

---

5. *Regimen of Health* 1:1.

> the organs obtain nourishment from any element in the food that is beneficial and whatever is unhealthy is expelled from the body. In this case, either no harm occurs or the harm that develops is not recognizable. However, overeating even the best foods can never, ever result in good digestion.[6]

We can conclude from Rambam that when it comes to diet, the primary concern must be quantity. The quality of food is of secondary concern.

Exercise

Regarding exercise, Rambam writes:

> A person who customarily exercises before meals does not have to be as careful (with his diet).[7]

It is not unusual to find people who overeat healthy foods and rarely exercise who are in much worse shape than people who exercise and eat lesser quality foods within reason.

What about waste management? Why is it left off Rambam's (and Hippocrates') primary list?

Rambam writes:

> This is a fundamental principle in medicine: When one is constipated or has difficulty moving his bowels, illness is approaching.[8]

Perhaps Rambam means to point out that problems with waste management are an indication rather than a direct cause of an inner imbalance which can lead to illness.

---

6. Ibid.
7. *Medical Aphorisms* 18:1.
8. *Mishneh Torah, Hilchos De'os* 4:13.

Obviously, it follows that if you are healthy internally, you will not experience problems with waste management. Therefore, it must be considered a passive principle, because if we follow the other main principles we can expect the elimination processes of our bodies to function efficiently. In fact, many people who formerly experienced problems in this area have seen significant improvements after beginning the Life-Transforming Diet.

TO SUM UP	
Primary Principle:	Food quantity
Primary Principle:	Exercise
Secondary Principle:	Food quality
Passive Principle:	Waste Management

Magic Formula

It seems that if we keep both the primary principles of Food Quantity and Exercise, it will create a compound which is greater than the sum of its parts. In other words, the combination of both primary principles creates a type of magic formula.

I think this explains a difficulty in the above Rambam. First, Rambam writes that a person will be healthy if he exercises, does not overeat and has loose bowels, "even if bad foods are eaten." Yet this is immediately followed by, "Most illnesses are caused by unhealthy foods." Rambam's first assertion seems to indicate that "bad foods" are of no concern to us, whereas his second statement seems to be saying that bad foods are one of the main causes of illness! (Clearly, Rambam is not talking about overeating bad foods, because he explicitly states that overeating even good foods is unhealthy!)

Therefore, I think Rambam is teaching us this wonderful insight: If we do not pay attention to both quantity of food and exercise, eating unhealthy foods will eventually lead to illness. We see this from Rambam's choice of words. He simply could have said that undereating bad foods will not harm our health. Instead, he says that if we watch quantity of food and exercise, we will be healthy and energetic *even if* we eat bad foods. It is specifically the synergy that is created by keeping both primary principles which results in the phenomenon of what I call the Magic Formula.

Now, this certainly doesn't mean that food quality is unimportant. After all, Rambam states explicitly that it is important. However, we are being told that if we eat the right amount of food and we exercise, then we do not have to be as concerned with the quality of food.

This dichotomy perplexed me for a long time. In fact, it took me a few years to truly internalize this observable reality. My problem was not the profound complexity of what Rambam was saying, but rather my preconceived perceptions which were blinding me from accepting the truth. I was misled because most health and weight programs are almost completely about *what* to eat, and that is what we have come to expect from any eating system. However, Rambam is teaching us that beneficial eating and lifestyle habits should take precedence.

TIMELESS PRINCIPLES

This is what I meant in the Introduction when I said that true principles are timeless and unchanging, whereas specific advice or theories may be disproved over time. Rambam's main principles of health are timeless. For example, overeating was, is and always will be, unhealthy for human beings because we were designed to hold and assimilate a certain quantity of food. Exercise was, is and always will be, a cornerstone of health because our bodies were designed so that we need to vigorously use each organ. Efficient bowel movements were, are and always will be, a fundamental aspect of health because we need to remove waste and toxins from the body. This is why Rambam uses the word Principle[9] when he talks about these aspects of health.

However, when it comes to specific food and nutritional suggestions, Rambam does not mention the term Principle. While he had clear opinions, they cannot be called Principles. I will elaborate why I think this is so.

Conflicting nutritional reports from the biggest news agencies in the world are an everyday occurrence. For instance, most of us are convinced that chocolate and coffee are very unhealthy. Yet I read one article that suggested that eating dark chocolate could help control diabetes and blood pressure.[10] Another article maintains that antioxidants in chocolate may increase "good" (HDL) cholesterol levels by as much as 10 percent. Regarding coffee, one article wrote how coffee not only helps clear the mind and raise energy levels, it also provides more healthful antioxidants than any other food or beverage in the American diet. Another article cites many benefits of coffee: It contains tannin and antioxidants, which are good for the heart and arteries. It can relieve headaches. It is good for the liver, and can help prevent cirrhosis and gallstones. And the caffeine in coffee can reduce the risk of asthma attacks and help improve circulation within the heart.

Regarding artificial sweeteners such as aspartame (i.e. NutraSweet and Equal), one article mentioned a new study suggesting a possible link between the artificial sweetener and brain tumors. But another article

9. *Mishneh Torah, Hilchos De'os* 4:15.
10. For Internet references supporting this and the following assertions, please see Appendix E on page 323.

states that the Food and Drug Administration said both it and the National Cancer Institute have found "no association between aspartame consumption and human brain tumors."

There are so many more examples of conflicting nutritional articles and news. As you can see, if we had to follow every new specific recommendation, we would have to change our diet almost every day!

Sometimes there are valid reasons why specific nutritional advice may change over time. In his *Regimen of Health*, Rambam writes regarding one of his specific food suggestions:

> People should not find it difficult or contradictory that many people eat this food and do not suffer from fever, because customs and predispositions [will cause reactions different from the norm]. For example, a Hindu would definitely get ill if he ate properly prepared bread and sheep's meat. Likewise, if one of us would constantly eat rice and fish as the Hindus always do, we would certainly get ill.[11]

In the introduction to his *Peirush HaMishnayos*, Rambam writes another possible reason:

> In each generation, extremely beneficial herbs and fruits are discovered that were not known to earlier generations. The human mind cannot grasp the advantages of each plant, but their benefits will become known through scientific experiment in time to come.

For all these reasons, I think the term Principle cannot be used when it comes to specific food and nutritional suggestions. This does not mean that we should ignore specific nutritional advice. But ultimately the truth of a system lies in its main principles and their effectiveness – principles

---

11. *Regimen of Health* 1:13.

which are logical, healthy practices, applicable in every time and in every circumstance. The key is to follow the principles and build from there, implementing specific nutritional advice based on the best available information.

Consequently, Rambam's primary principles of Food Quantity and Exercise play a central role in our system. Of course, food quality is also dealt with in detail, but it takes a secondary position in the practical day-to-day progression of the Phases.

RAMBAM'S FOUR MAIN INGREDIENTS FOR OPTIMUM HEALTH REVISITED

Food Quantity

Most people assume that the subject of food quantity applies only to how much food you eat at a meal. However, there are three different ways you can overeat:

1. Having too many meals
2. At a meal
3. Between meals

I will discuss each one of these types of overeating in detail, and present some practical methods for dealing with the challenge of overeating.

Exercise

The ancient physicians wrote about the three main components of an exercise program (cardio, strengthening and stretching). Rambam also stresses the psychosomatic component of exercising.

Continued on next page

You will learn how to implement a well-balanced, basic exercise program at the right pace. Obviously, you do not have to build up slowly if you are already following a well-balanced exercise program.

Food Quality

Amazingly, Rambam's extensive writings on refined and high-fat foods seem like they could have been written today. Beneficial foods, cuts of meat and methods of cooking are all discussed. Up-to-date, concise and to the point, Rambam's advice is easily substantiated by modern-day professionals.

Waste Management

Rambam teaches us how to insure that this bodily function runs smoothly.[12]

Above, we see in a few short lines how Rambam succeeds in laying down the foundation and sketching the outline for an effective system. It is from this nucleus that we will build a practical system incorporating Rambam's many works.

Obviously, a great deal of explanation of Rambam's principles is still required. Most important, we have to learn how to practically and comfortably implement these principles. And Rambam's works are filled with helpful, practical advice.

But first we must understand the mechanics of habit formation and list our incentives for making a life transformation.

---

12. See *Mishneh Torah, Hilchos De'os* 4:2, 14, 16; *Regimen of Health* 1:5.

INSIGHTS AND SUCCESS STORIES

Rachel from the United States lost 40 pounds – tried everything

You name the diet, I've probably tried it! Protein diets, food combining diets, appetite suppressants, and diet shakes. I've even had injections and gone on some really radical programs. Each diet had its positive aspects, but ultimately I felt bored and deprived by their monotonous repetitiveness. On some diets, I became a nervous wreck! I just could not continue after a while.

The Life-Transforming Diet has taught me how I can choose to eat.

I like to eat carbohydrates, combine different food groups and snack once in a while. I can do all this because I have worked through the Phases and I'm maintaining my goal weight according to plan. This program is about me and my choices, not rules and food restrictions.

After I worked through the Phases, I customized the program to suit my schedule and interests. I can't believe it; it's like a dream come true!

Tamar from the United States – Optimum health

I did not need to lose weight, but I wanted to develop better eating habits. I was feeling tired a lot of the time and my energy levels were very low. So I decided to give the Life-Transforming Diet a chance. Very soon, I realized how bad my eating habits had been. I was used to eating low-quality foods. Few of my meals were nutritious. Now, my perspective on food has changed and my eating habits have really changed for the better. I eat all my meals with confidence and I also enjoy making some Smart Exceptions. I weigh the same, but I am much fitter and I feel on top of the world.

CHAPTER 2
MIND GAMES

CREATURES OF HABIT

Often we really want to change; but why don't we?

We don't change because we are creatures of habit!

Rambam writes:

> One of the most powerful forces of human nature is habit,
> irrespective of whether these are actions or preconceived
> perceptions.... For instance, a person might choose bad foods
> to which he is accustomed over good foods to which he is not
> accustomed[1] [even though it is the less correct choice].

Let's look at the following scenarios:

- As a result of bad eating habits, someone suffers from heartburn every
  night. Before going to bed, he resolves to eat better the next day.

- Someone else weighs himself during the course of the day and gasps,
  "Wow, there must be something wrong with this scale!" After his wife
  assures him that it is in fact accurate, he resolves to eat better for the
  rest of the day.

The next day – or a few hours later – the cravings begin and old habits
creep back. At first, the people in these examples may resist, but eventually

---

1. *Treatise on Asthma* 13:51. See also *Moreh Nevuchim* 1:31.

they say to themselves, "What's the difference? Just one; one can't hurt." But soon, one becomes two, and before they know it, it's back to heartburn at night and "scale fright" in the morning.

What happened to that powerful moment of inspiration? To where did that firm resolve to eat better disappear? Surely the desire to prevent pain at night and anguish in the morning is greater than a few seconds of pleasure.[2] Perhaps because the pleasure is immediate, whereas the pain is out of sight for the moment, the animalistic pull for immediate satisfaction outweighs any potential or future discomfort. The "animal" mind does not weigh the consequences of its actions.

And what about the person who continues to eat badly, even though he suffers from heartburn right now? What about people with severe health problems who continue to eat unhealthily despite the pain or the very real possibility of a fatal attack?

The same situation applies to smokers. There are many well-known cases of patients who continue to smoke in spite of cancer or amputated limbs!

The weaker will to enjoy a few seconds of pleasure overpowers the stronger will to prevent instantaneous pain. How?

Let's look at how habits play with our minds.

2. See *Michtav Me'Eliyahu*, vol. 1, "Free Choice," p. 111, which brings out a different point from a very similar case.

S.A.P. – SUBCONSCIOUS ACCUMULATION PROCESS

This is possibly one of the most exciting subjects I have ever come across. I sincerely believe that after reading this chapter, you will never look at the world in the same way again!

Many programs designed to "break bad habits" do not even discuss how habits are formed in the first place. They merely state that habits become second nature.

Let me begin by asking a simple question: In terms of character development, what is more significant – giving one dollar each to one thousand charities, or giving a thousand dollars to one charity? In the first case, many people gain but the overall impact is minor. In the second case, only a single significant donation is made but it can go a long way to help. Is one better than the other? Or is each one equally positive?

Rambam writes:

> Positive behavior characteristics are not acquired by doing great (positive) acts but rather *through the repetition of many positive acts*. For example, giving a thousand gold coins to one charity will not accustom a person to the trait of generosity, whereas giving one gold coin to a thousand different charities will do so. By repeating an act many times, an established behavior or emotional pattern is formed. In contrast, one great act represents an arousal to good, after which that motivation may disappear.[3]

Rambam is teaching us a fundamental principle in human nature. Even a simple habit can have more of an impact on our personal development than a major motivational arousal! But why is habit so much more

---

3. Commentary on *Pirkei Avos* 3:18.

powerful? What is the difference between the first, second and third time we do something?[4] After all, it is exactly the same act repeated over and over again. The answer is that real change takes place *within*, not without. I like to call this the Subconscious Accumulation Process, or S.A.P.

In the early 1800s, some of our greatest authorities[5] explained how habits are formed. This is the essence of what they wrote:

> Learning a new language is a good analogy [of habit formation]. In order for the student to learn how to pronounce words, the teacher must first expend a great deal of effort and skill in order to teach him the different letters of the alphabet. Then he learns how to join the letters together to form words. He must work extremely hard to learn this skill. *Eventually, however, through habit, this skill becomes a function of the subconscious*, and he learns to read with ease and without conscious effort.
>
> We can apply this same process to the realm of emotions. There are both conscious and subconscious factors [in habit formation].[6]

> Every single feeling, no matter how small it is and even if it is forgotten immediately by the conscious mind, always leaves some sort of impression on the memory. If one then experiences this feeling a second time, it combines with the original impression, thereby strengthening itself. Every time this feeling is experienced again, *all the accumulated traces of the previous impressions combine with it.*

---

4. See *Mishneh Torah, Hilchos De'os* 1:7.
5. Rav Yisrael Salanter, who quotes *Cheshbon HaNefesh* as a source regarding this subject.
6. *Ohr Yisrael*, Letter 6.

From here we can understand how *the power of habit strengthens even the weakest feelings*, and how it creates learned desires which intensify over time.[7]

Over time, the most insignificant string of experiences can accumulate to become strong enough to overwhelm even a major experience.[8]

This is the power of habit!

The outer action may be exactly the same every time you repeat it, but the subconscious accumulation of every minor experience, feeling and image associated with that act gains more momentum each time it is repeated.

When we understand this mechanism, then every experience, feeling and image takes on a new meaning. In fact, this inner process affects every aspect of our personalities and behavior.

HABIT'S EXPLOSIVE EFFECT

The Talmud says that you cannot compare someone who learned something 100 times to someone who learned something 101 times.[9] He who learned it 101 times is considered to be on a much more advanced level. Why? Is there really such a difference between 100 times and 101 times?

The answer is Absolutely!

---

7. See *Cheshbon HaNefesh* 53.
8. See ibid., 55.
9. *Chagigah* 9b. This was said regarding intellectual pursuits, but we saw above that the same applies to emotional development. See also *Ohr Yisrael*, Letter 6.

Let us assume that you have the exact same experience 101 times. Each experience leaves the same one impression on your mind. So you would think that the difference between the hundredth experience and the hundred-and-first experience is still only one impression. However, this is only true if there is no link between the different experiences.

This is where the accumulation process changes everything.

As we said above, every single experience, even if "forgotten" by the conscious mind, always leaves some sort of impression on the memory. Every time the experience is repeated, the original experience is revived and reinforced. All traces of the previous impressions accumulate.

In other words, you may have exactly the same experience each time, but the impressions or traces left on your memory are much more significant each time it is repeated. These impressions accumulate and snowball over time because each new experience encapsulates all the previous experiences.

Therefore, even though there is just one external *experience* which separates the hundredth time and hundred-and-first time, internally there is a difference of possibly 101 *impressions* – the 100 previous impressions plus the current impression. There is certainly not just one impression's difference between the hundredth and the hundred-and-first times![10]

Now, what happens if the accumulation of traces is not simply a linear accumulation? What happens if the experiences compound over time? If the impressions retain their impact over time, then the difference between the hundredth time and the hundred-and-first time could be as many as 5151 impressions!

10. While it is definitely possible that the impact of earlier impressions decrease over time, there is always some sort of trace which remains. These traces are then carried over to any future similar experiences.

THE POWER OF SUBCONSCIOUS ACCUMULATION

1st experience		= 1 impression
2nd experience	This impression 2 + previous impression 1	= 3 impressions
3rd experience	This impression 3 + previous impressions 3	= 6 impressions
4th experience	This impression 4 + previous impressions 6	= 10 impressions
5th experience	This impression 5 + previous impressions 10	= 15 impressions
6th experience	This impression 6 + previous impressions 15	= 21 impressions...
99th experience	This impression 99 + previous impressions 4851	= 4950 impressions
100th experience	This impression 100 + previous impressions 4950	= 5050 impressions
101st experience	This impression 101 + previous impressions 5050	= 5151 impressions

No matter how you slice it, it is clear that habits are the result of a very powerful Subconscious Accumulation Process. After sufficient repetitions, we probably experience a colossal emotional explosion every time we have the same experience or do the same exact act!

In light of this, we can now appreciate the above statement from the Talmud. One more experience certainly *does* make a world of difference.

It is virtually impossible to conceptualize what goes on in our brains every single minute! It has rightfully been said, "No computer has yet come close to the brain" (*Merck Manual*, 1987).

The "accumulation of traces" concept also explains why big companies are prepared to spend millions of dollars on constant advertising. It is not just about providing a repetitive information service: advertisements really do play with our minds! We are usually not even aware of the images and feelings that have accumulated in our subconscious as a result of the repeated messages. Constant flashy food advertisements have certainly contributed to the obesity epidemic!

Only someone who is "addicted" can truly appreciate the extreme accumulation of impressions he experiences in every fiber of his being! This applies to food, drink, smoking or any other activity, thought or feeling to which there is an "addiction." The addicted individual experiences a virtual explosion of traces and impressions left on his psyche.

Now we can understand how a weaker will to enjoy a few seconds of smoking is able to overcome the stronger will to prevent pain. A non-smoker will look at the smoker and wonder how he can make such seemingly illogical decisions. The former has clarity of vision because he is psychologically sober about the hazards of smoking cigarettes. The smoker, however, is trapped in the clutches of a habit which he himself originally set in motion. The phenomenal accumulation of feelings, images and experiences compel him to smoke even in the face of any logical reason why he should not. The same applies to the person who continues to eat badly even though he knows all too well that he will regret it later that night or the next morning.

It isn't difficult to see the manifestation of the Subconscious Accumulation Process in our constant encounters with food and in our eating habits. What may start off as simple acts, whether overindulgence in or unhealthy abstention from food, can become obsessive eating disorders through habit. Eventually, all traces of experiences, feelings and images that are associated with food and eating habits accumulate to form extremely powerful inner motivational forces.

THE FOOD CONNECTION

The following example illustrates very clearly the interaction between the Subconscious Accumulation Process and our eating habits.

Imagine a thick piece of creamy delicious chocolate cake with warm icing melting over its edges. (Perhaps an even better example is the prospect of taking a second helping after finishing a satisfying meal.) What goes on inside your head?

You hear one voice which says, "Mmm, I really want to eat this! I love chocolate cake and this looks irresistibly delicious. It's my favorite food, I really want another helping. No one is looking…"

Then suddenly, just before you reach out to take a second helping, a small voice interjects, "But you know you really shouldn't. You'll feel guilty later on. You'll be sorry!"

We can all relate to this very common experience. Let's take a few moments to carefully analyze the above inner debate and you will notice something absolutely fascinating.

The voice which tempts you to eat the cake or take another helping is in the first person: *I* want to eat it; *I* love this food. In contrast, the "responsible" voice is in the second person: *You* know that you will regret this; *You* know you shouldn't.

The voice that speaks to us in the first person is our first instinctive natural response. In contrast, the "logical voice" speaks to us in the second person, which makes it further removed. It is almost as if another person is talking to us.[11] Therefore, if there is a clash between the "I" and the "You" responses, the You stands very little chance.

Thus, it seems that there is some validity to the popular justification: "I have very little willpower. I just can't control myself or my cravings!" Willpower alone is in fact weaker than a craving or a bad eating habit. Unfortunately, most of us know this from bitter experience. But how can we change the tide?

Through the Subconscious Accumulation Process!

It is definitely possible to accumulate traces of willpower until there is enough momentum to overcome even the most powerful cravings or entrenched bad habits. The Subconscious Accumulation Process can develop a small spark of inspiration into a burning flame of motivation and eventually transformation.

Now let us return to *Cheshbon HaNefesh* and understand its profound ramifications:

> The sheer strength of "willpower" is inconsequential when compared to an intense desire. [Willpower is desire governed by the intellect.] As a result, if there is a sudden confrontation between these two forces, willpower will be overcome easily.
>
> Nevertheless, due to the kindness of our Creator, the small impressions of willpower are not eliminated completely. Instead, they constantly leave traces which, over time, accumulate so that eventually the strength of willpower increases enough to

11. See *Nefesh HaChaim* 1:6. See also *Michtav Me'Eliyahu*, vol. 2, *Parashas Bereishis*, p. 138.

> overwhelm even the most intense desires [or motivations] through this Divine assistance.[12]

Even the most entrenched habits, addictions and cravings can be overcome by new accumulated motivations, although initially they are much weaker. By implementing a new habit at the right pace, old entrenched desires start to fade. Old habits are slowly replaced by new ones. Eventually, a real change can and will take place.

TRANSFORMATION

At the point of change, you will not simply be *overcoming* your nature. You will start to experience a strong urge to follow beneficial eating and lifestyle habits – you will *want* to make the right choices.[13] In terms of our previous example, the "I" and the "You" will switch positions. Now the responsible voice becomes the "I": "*I* don't want to eat that doughnut or do that thing." The voice which tempts becomes the "You": "*You* know that used to be your favorite." You still experience temptation, but it is the weaker will and it is external.

At the ultimate level of transformation, you are no longer making the correct choices with your intellect; you are making them reflexively. In effect, your "Reactive Mind" stays exactly the same – shortsighted and impulsive. However, now the source of your particular motivation is healthy. This is the direct result of a *perception change*, which I will discuss in more detail in Chapter 12. So you still react automatically, but now it is in accordance with these positive, inner motivations.

12. See *Cheshbon HaNefesh* 56.
13. See *Ohr Yisrael*, Letter 17; *Moreh Nevuchim* 1:2; *Sifsei Chaim, Middos v'Avodas Hashem,* Modesty 9.

Rabbi Yisrael Salanter says that character improvement begins with *controlling* or restraining an inner urge. Eventually a person can reach the level of actually *transforming* an urge so that no *inner* conflict is experienced at all.[14] In *Shemoneh Perakim*,[15] Rambam mentions these two levels of character development.[16] Rambam refers to the first level of Control as "ruling over his spirit" and the second, higher level of Transformation as "piety."

A transformation or "perception change" is the most effective way to deal with a bad habit because it prevents or removes it at its source. This is the opposite of repressing a feeling, thought or action, which is bound to manifest itself in other ways – probably leading to rebellion or despair.

Now we can understand and truly appreciate why Rambam calls his famous section on character traits and emotions *Hilchos De'os*, "The Laws of Perceptions."[17]

I think this also explains why Rambam places his health and eating advice in this same section. It is pointless to try simply to change external bad eating habits. As Rambam writes, "Many of our bad food choices and bad eating habits originate from our trained perceptions."[18]

Think about these concepts deeply. They apply to every situation in life.

A transformation is fascinating and exciting. It is the ultimate stage of change. The Life-Transforming Diet offers a precise plan of action which will unleash the power of the Subconscious Accumulation Process.

You are on the way to transforming yourself!

---

14. *Ohr Yisrael*, Letter 30.
15. Chapter 6.
16. He writes this regarding the "rational commandments." See *Ohr Yisrael*, Letter 30, for a detailed discussion on this section of Rambam.
17. *Hilchos De'os* is sometimes misleadingly translated as "The Laws of Temperaments."
18. *Treatise on Asthma* 13:51.

INSIGHTS AND SUCCESS STORIES

Osnat from South Africa lost over 60 pounds in six months using S.A.P.

What makes this diet different from every other diet I have endured? I think it is the brilliance of using the Subconscious Accumulation Process to form new positive habits in order to fight the old established ones. I didn't have to eliminate everything in one go.

The emphasis in the Life-Transforming Diet is not on "willpower"; the focus is rather on the gradual development of good habits. It is so clever to slowly cultivate positive habits and to help them grow until they are big enough and strong enough to dissolve the former "monster" habits. Becoming aware of the ability of my "creative mind" to make decisions has been very enlightening, and I have never been so calm about food and food choices. I don't feel like indulging in any of my old temptations, and I'm not waiting for the opportunity to "break out." I haven't felt deprived or trapped – in fact, I feel energized!

Yaakov from Israel – Beyond the External

I have been studying in yeshiva full-time for many years and I always thought that health and nutrition were for people who were into external appearances. I never realized that being overweight is a very real medical risk. I was intrigued that our eating habits involve some of the most complex aspects of our thought processes and often have very little to do with the food itself. This subject should be mastered by everyone.

CHAPTER 3
PRACTICALLY SPEAKING

COMPARING OTHER DIETS

If you compare this program to other popular diets, you will find that this program has much more flexibility and more food choices while offering a balanced, nutritious diet. My intention here is not to bash other diets but to prove this point. Let me show you very briefly.

Government Nutritional Information

The problem is that we are bombarded with too much information. This necessitates copious sorting of information and then we are left without a method for actually implementing this information. Furthermore, some of the suggested quantities seem to be over-exaggerated.

No-Carb Diets

Fruit, vegetables and grains are entirely eliminated. High in saturated fats and low in fiber foods, this diet is not healthy nor is it practical in the long term.

Low-Carb Diets

This is really a modified no-carb diet. Excessive protein is still recommended at the meals and between meals while the consumption of fruits and grains is forbidden. The change is that now there is an allowance for the very controlled consumption of these healthy foods at later stages of the diet. The problem is the quantities of these foods are small and most low-carb dieters never actually reach that "later Phase." This is not surprising because the majority of the weight loss is achieved during the first stage when fruits and grains are restricted entirely. But since these restrictions cannot be maintained long-term, it is not long before the dieter gives up and returns to his old eating habits.

Low-Fat, High-Carb Diets

These diets have the opposite difficulty. Can you really eliminate flesh proteins from your diet? Some of these diets also demand total fat restriction. This means that you will not be getting your necessary fat-soluble vitamins or essential fatty acids. Furthermore, fat-free low-quality snacks which are high in refined flour, sugar, preservatives and calories are often overeaten. After all, it's still fat-free!

Naturopathic or Natural Hygiene Diets

Here it is forbidden to combine protein and starches in one meal. You can never eat a protein sandwich or chicken and potatoes together again! Furthermore, these diets also severely limit the *quantities* of protein. Eggs, fish, chicken and yogurt must be limited to once or twice a week in small quantities. Milk and red meat are even more restricted.

Calorie-Counting or Food-Measuring Diets

These systems are simply too time-consuming and involved. Count or weigh everything! Very often this leads to obsessive eating habits or general food obsession. Furthermore, calories take precedence over nutritious healthy foods. The Glycemic Index (GI) diets have a similar problem. For example, potato chips have a lower GI score than do watermelon or brown rice.

Every one of these diets has some excellent aspects, but in practice long-term observance is almost impossible to sustain and in many cases the diets are unhealthy. Hence the never-ending search for the perfect solution – the new fad diet that promises to deliver that much-coveted dream of "normal weight."

So, you may be wondering, what is different about the Life-Transforming Diet? What distinguishes our program from all these other popular regimes?

The Life-Transforming Diet, based on the principles of Rambam, is a program that can be realistically sustained. We restrict neither food quantities nor any type of nutritious foods. We propose eating principles. You can choose which nutritious foods to eat when implementing these positive eating habits.

In addition, the Life-Transforming Diet develops an awareness of habit formation and implements behavior modification, which increases self-awareness on a motivational and behavioral level. This is fundamental to the success of the program and clearly distinguishes it from other systems. It is not a diet that gives you a definitive list of what you can eat, what you cannot eat and what exact amounts you are limited to have.

The Life-Transforming Diet is a method of understanding not only what to eat but *how* to eat, with an explanation of inner motivational forces as well as external behavior patterns. If you follow the principles then you do not have to weigh, count or restrict your food. All of this is explained in detail in the book.

Interestingly, many of the positive attributes of each of the above-mentioned diets are found in the Life-Transforming Diet. Ours is a workable, realistic system that allows you to go on living your own particular lifestyle while you gradually transform your life.

AN OVERVIEW OF OUR PRACTICAL NUTRITIONAL PRINCIPLES

At a great risk of oversimplification of our nutritional principles, I will briefly show you what to expect. All the theory, particulars and daily examples will be discussed in detail throughout the book, but these are the main principles as they manifest in everyday life.

High Water Content (HWC) Meal

This meal is an easy-to-digest, cleansing and, as the name suggests, mostly high-water-content meal. There are two choices. The first is a large bowl of fruit or mixed fruit platter. A topping of nuts may be added. The second is a large salad with a nonfat, low-fat or homemade dressing. Some people like to start with a vegetable soup. Medium-starchy vegetables such as carrots, butternut squash, pumpkin or beets and a topping of seeds such as sunflower seeds may also be eaten with this mostly vegetable meal. Although the nuts and seeds are restricted, the fruits and vegetables are not.

One-Concentrated-Food (One CF) Meal

Here there are two choices as well. You may have either protein with vegetables or starch with vegetables. For instance, instead of steak with potatoes, you would replace the potatoes with grilled vegetables or the steak with grilled vegetables. Instead of fish with couscous, you could replace either the couscous or the fish with steamed vegetables.

A lighter version of this meal consists of eating a protein topping on a salad or eating starches such as bread, potatoes or pasta. Bread can be eaten as a sandwich with vegetables or together with a salad. The same applies to potato. Pasta (preferably whole wheat) can be eaten with marinara sauce.

Portions are not restricted at One-Concentrated-Food meals.

Mixed Meal

Your other meal can consist of both protein and starch, but only take seconds of the vegetables. Thus, you can eat a meat sandwich or chicken with potatoes. Cereal with milk is another option. But if you are hungry after eating your usual portion, only take seconds of salad and/or cut up vegetables and not of the concentrated foods.

Substitution between Meals

We will encourage drinking and eating vegetables, fruit or low-fat dairy products between meals.

Ultimately, there will also be other snacks allowed between meals, even the less nutritious ones, within the guidelines of "Smart Exceptions." Dessert options will change through the Phases of this diet.

PRACTICAL IMPLEMENTATION

This is where this program shines! Based on Rambam's opinion regarding changing habits, we will implement the above principles at the right pace.

We will introduce *only one* change every week.

In the first week, it is the HWC meal.

In the second week, we add a five- to ten-minute exercise workout. If you are already following a balanced exercise program, you can continue with what you are doing.

In the third week, we will introduce Substitution between Meals.

The fourth week introduces the main version of the One CF Meal.

In the fifth week, we will add the lighter version of the One CF Meal.

This ends Phase 1.

Phase 2 is simply a continuation of Phase 1. The only thing that will change is your exercise program. Otherwise you will simply continue with the guidelines of Phase 1 for three weeks. Many people lose five to ten pounds in this Phase alone.

In Phase 3, we introduce the Mixed Meal and more dessert options. You will continue in this Phase until you are at your goal weight. At that point, you will be allowed more snack options between meals as well as dessert options called Smart Exceptions.

It's that simple and that quick!

The relevant chapters detail a clear, practical implementation of our principles. You will also learn how to deal practically with "excursions" – deviations from the program. Excursions are an expected part of this journey, and you will learn how to get back on track and how to make up for any lost ground.

A very simple Personal Ledger system will also be introduced, which is based on the teachings of our great Mussar teachers. In our Ledgers, you will simply have to write a number in a box.

As you can see, this program deals with both the practical and the psychological aspects of behavior modification.

A NUTRITIONAL PERSPECTIVE

It should be clear why our way of eating does not over-restrict the amount of calories consumed, because we encourage all the main nutritious foods and are very liberal with our food quantities.

First, we do not limit fruit and vegetable consumption. Second, we do not even limit the amount you eat of a concentrated food when you follow the guidelines of the One CF Meal. For example, you are not limited to a 3-ounce piece of chicken. You are allowed to eat any amount of chicken, and you can take more helpings of it, provided that you do not walk away from the meal feeling sick. If you are eating bread as your one concentrated food, you could take more portions of bread. The same applies to potatoes, pasta or any other starch. Sometimes it is necessary to do this because years of deprivation and starvation in an attempt to shed weight causes anxiety. After a while, when you realize that no one is restricting you, you will become aware of your own natural appetite and the quantities of food will diminish accordingly.

You may say that requiring no set food quantities is a contradiction of Rambam's principle of quantity. Good question, but the answer is that you will soon learn about the beauty of the One CF Meal. It has the digestive advantages that allow you eventually to *naturally* stop at the point you personally need to stop. Hard to believe, I know, but this has been verified by so many people on this system that we know it's true. As Rambam says, everyone should determine his own personal quantity of food intake.[1] This will be done naturally once you have reinstated the integrity of your body's appetite control system.

A Mixed Meal does not have these digestive advantages, so at this meal you will only take seconds of vegetables. However, make sure to eat a

---

1.   *Treatise on Asthma* 5:1. See also *Commentary on Hippocrates' Aphorisms* 1:17. The full quote from Rambam is found on page 141 of this book.

moderate, satisfying portion of protein and starch. Just use common sense. The Mixed Meal has more food combination options, but since it lacks the advantages of the One CF Meal and requires a bit more "self control," we only add it in Phase 3. Put into context, you could be going without a Mixed Meal for as little as four weeks.

As you can see, the Life-Transforming Diet has so many options. Our system is not about restrictions, practically or psychologically. It's about gaining balanced nutritional information and implementing it through a practical system which allows for a lot of flexibility and personal customization. It allows you to have a "mature" relationship with food.

I am truly excited for you because you are about to transform your life, your perspectives on food and your eating habits. Your friends and family will soon share your excitement as they witness the transformation. Please let us know about your success. (See page 257, footnote 11, for our contact information.)

INSIGHTS AND SUCCESS STORIES

Sheindy from South Africa – "A truly life-transforming program"

The Life-Transforming Diet is nothing less than...life-transforming. I began the diet somewhat skeptical (after many unsuccessful attempts at unsustainable diets). But I quickly became a believer and possibly even a groupie! The Phases are brilliantly structured in a way that makes them easy to begin and easy to sustain. Already in the few weeks I have been on the program I have seen and felt a remarkable difference in my energy levels, my food choices and my (lack of) cravings. I feel empowered, understanding the reasons behind healthy choices, as opposed to just being handed a list of what's taboo. My friends and family tell me I am glowing. This program is truly life-transforming because it hasn't just affected my way of eating and viewing food but it has affected every single aspect of my life. I feel more disciplined, more motivated and totally liberated.

CHAPTER 4
WHY SHOULD I CHANGE?

INCENTIVES

Rambam writes:

> Human nature is incentive-based.[1]

Why are incentives so important?

Human nature refuses to make changes if the new choice provides less enjoyment or causes more distress than the current situation. However, if a new practice or way of life is theoretically less enjoyable but practically will provide a greater advantage, we will *want* to change. Notice that we have shifted our personal definition of the "greater enjoyment" or the "lesser distress" to be in line with the "greater advantage." This way, we are working *with* human nature, rather than against it.

The goal of gaining health and losing weight evokes many general incentives. However, their very generality makes them fuzzy and difficult to define, and does not lead to significant results. It is important to zero in on some specific personal incentives. Furthermore, a clear understanding of our incentives will also help us to accept the short-term discomfort that invariably accompanies making any real change.

In his *Moreh Nevuchim*,[2] Rambam lists four categories of general human accomplishment: External possessions, physical health and strength, moral

---

1. Introduction to *Perek Chelek*.
2. 3:54.

virtues, and rational virtues – specifically regarding knowledge of God. Together, these categories represent ultimate human perfection. I think that there are four similar incentives that should constantly motivate us to gain health and lose weight permanently:[3]

1. EXTERNAL APPEARANCE

Most of us spend a considerable amount of time, money and effort trying to improve our external appearance. After all, who doesn't want to look good? We all want to fit into normal-size clothing, and nobody wants to be a "slob." The dating scene really highlights this issue. The inevitable question is always, "What does she look like?" Likewise, obese children are teased at school, and insensitive comments continue to plague them into adolescence and adulthood.

As people mature, the snide remarks and attitudes are disguised in more subtle packages. For instance, statistics show that it is much harder for an obese person to get a job. Of course, we should have a non-judgmental perception of others, but whether we like it or not, most people *do* "judge a book by its cover." It is therefore no surprise that the beauty, fitness and weight-loss industry is one of the biggest and fastest-growing today.

Rambam writes that the Torah took this aspect of human nature into account:

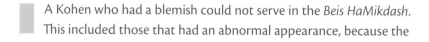 A Kohen who had a blemish could not serve in the *Beis HaMikdash*. This included those that had an abnormal appearance, because the

---

3. A similar concept of different levels of incentive is listed in *Mesillas Yesharim*, Chapter 4, concerning acquiring *zehirus* (vigilance).

> multitude does not evaluate an individual by his true form [i.e. his intellect], but by the *perfection of his body and the beauty of his clothes.*[4]

Thus, concern for external appearances can be a very powerful incentive for making lifestyle changes. In fact, according to many Torah Sources, we are expected to look presentable, neat[5] and pleasant[6] in appearance.

2. OPTIMUM HEALTH AND DISEASE PREVENTION

Rambam stresses the importance of directing our actions for the sake of health:

> Whether a person eats, drinks, has marital relations, sleeps, is awake, performs activities or rests, the primary goal should be to preserve his physical health.[7]

Nowadays, because of increased public awareness, improvement of health has become a popular incentive for making lifestyle changes. For one thing, an unhealthy lifestyle causes health problems. Being overweight or obese not only disfigures a person physically and psychologically, but most important − it is a very real medical risk. There is no way to dress it up: *excess weight is simply dangerous.*

According to the National Institutes of Health,[8] people who are classified as overweight are considered at risk for premature death and disability.

---

4. *Moreh Nevuchim* 3:45.
5. See *Mishneh Torah, Hilchos De'os* 5:1,9.
6. Rashi, *Devarim* 14:1.
7. *Shemoneh Perakim*, Chapter 5.
8. National Institutes of Health, "Clinical Guidelines on the Identification, Evaluation, and Treatment of Overweight and Obesity in Adults." Bethesda, Maryland: Department

In fact, did you know that excess weight may have even more negative health consequences than smoking or drinking? Two researchers for Rand Health Publications, health economist Roland Sturm and psychiatrist Kenneth Wells, examined the comparative effects of obesity, smoking, heavy drinking, and poverty on chronic health conditions and health expenditures. Their finding: *Obesity is the most serious problem*. It is linked to a big increase in chronic health conditions and significantly higher health expenditures. Not only does obesity have more negative health consequences than smoking, drinking, or poverty, it also affects more people.[9]

Many people are simply unaware of the many health problems that are likely to develop from being overweight. One of the most common and serious diseases which can result from being overweight is type 2 diabetes. In fact, overweight people are more than fifteen times more likely to develop the condition than those of normal weight, and obese people are twenty to fifty times more likely to do so.[10]

Can we really prevent type 2 diabetes through better diet and lifestyle habits? The answer is Yes. Even those medical professionals who believe that genetics plays an important role in type 2 diabetes maintain that this is just a predisposition. Even more astounding is that following a healthy regimen can help in treating and perhaps even removing an existing condition.

The following survey really helps put things into clear perspective. In 2002, the Diabetes Prevention Program (DPP) conducted a major clinical trial

of Health and Human Services, National Institutes of Health, National Heart, Lung, and Blood Institute, 1998.
9.   For Internet references backing up this and the following facts and statistics, please see Appendix E on page 323.
10. From Harvard Health Publications, *Weigh Less, Live Longer: Strategies for Successful Weight Loss*. Cambridge, MA: President and Fellows of Harvard College, 2004.

with more than 3000 people who had impaired glucose tolerance. This is a condition that often precedes diabetes. All of the people were also overweight. The study consisted of three different groups of people:

1. One group made intensive lifestyle changes including diet and exercise.

2. Another group was treated with the oral diabetes drug metformin.

3. A control group was given a placebo in place of metformin. (The second and third groups also received standard information on diet and exercise.)

On the advice of the DPP's external data monitoring board, the trial ended a year early because the data had clearly answered the main research questions.

During the average follow-up period of three years, about 29 percent of the DPP group taking the placebo developed diabetes. Twenty-two percent of the metformin group developed diabetes. The diet and exercise group had the best results, with only 14 percent developing diabetes.

Here is a list of other health problems associated with being overweight, recorded by the National Institutes of Health:[11]

- Coronary heart disease

- Angina pectoris

- High blood pressure, hypertension

- High blood cholesterol, dyslipidemia[12]

11. "Clinical Guidelines on the Identification, Evaluation, and Treatment of Overweight and Obesity in Adults," pp. 12–20.
12. Dyslipidemia is a disruption in the amount of lipids in the blood. (Lipids are a class of hydrocarbon-containing organic compounds essential for the structure and function of living cells.)

- Congestive heart failure

- Cancer (such as endometrial, breast, prostate, and colon). While tobacco is linked to about 30 percent of cancer cases, diet is involved in an estimated 25 percent of cases.[13]

- Stroke

- Insulin resistance, glucose intolerance

- Hyperinsulinemia[14]

- Gallstones

- Gout

- Osteoarthritis

- Obstructive sleep apnea and respiratory problems

- Complications during pregnancy

- Poor female reproductive health (such as menstrual irregularities, infertility, irregular ovulation)

- Bladder control problems (such as stress incontinence)

- Uric acid nephrolithiasis[15]

This list is no exaggeration! Take a look at life insurance premiums. The more you weigh the greater your life insurance premiums are, even if you are otherwise in "perfect health." To make matters worse, many companies refuse to insure someone who is extremely overweight.

---

13. Patricia Reaney, "Diet, Alcohol Linked to Nearly One Third of Cancer Cases" (Reuters-Health, 2004).
14. Hyperinsulinemia means you have too much insulin in your blood. It isn't diabetes, but it is often associated with type 2 diabetes.
15. The formation of crystal aggregates in the urinary tract, resulting in kidney stones.

The health consequences of being obese or overweight are certainly not a new discovery. Rambam writes:

> Obesity is harmful to the body: makes it lethargic, disturbs its functions and hampers its movements.[16]

> Someone who is healthy and of *intermediate body mass* is most likely to reach old age.[17]

However, do not be fooled that the diseases mentioned above are limited to people who are overweight. Though carrying extra weight increases the chances, unhealthy eating and lifestyle habits are main contributors to the development of disease *no matter how thin you look*! This is no longer just a claim made by the "alternative" medical associations. Look at all the main government conventional medical associations set up to research and combat the big killer diseases – heart disease, cancer, stroke and diabetes. They all give the same advice on how to prevent and reduce these fatal diseases: "Eat a healthier diet, exercise regularly, lose weight and put a stop to harmful habits that contribute to those diseases."

By improving your eating and lifestyle habits, you reduce the risk of incurring fatal diseases. In addition, you will notice that you become sick far less frequently and with much milder symptoms than before. Why should you feel tired, lethargic or out of breath? There is a wonderful, vibrant feeling that comes with being healthy. The body is injected with energy, a zest for life and a much better perspective of the world.

16. *Medical Aphorisms* 9:101.
17. *Commentary on Hippocrates' Aphorisms* 2:44.

Fear Factor

Contemplating the terrible diseases and loss of potential that can result from certain diets and lifestyle habits mobilizes an innate aspect of our natures. Our psyche is programmed so that fear of something removes the desire to do that which may lead to it.[18]

In many ways, fear is more effective than any intellectual argument. The reason for this is that the root of fear is found in our basic instincts. Like desire, it is implanted within every living creature. So even when the force of an instinct seems to overcome the intellect, one can arouse the trait of fear from the same source as the instinct.[19] This is a very important concept, and it has many ramifications.

What Constitutes Overweight?

In general, overweight is defined as one to thirty pounds over a healthy weight, and obesity is defined as being thirty pounds or more over a healthy weight. For a more precise measure, the Body Mass Index (BMI) is more highly correlated with body fat than any other indicator. BMI is a ratio which measures weight relative to height.

The definitions of "healthy weight," "overweight" and "obesity" were established after numerous studies took the BMIs of millions of people and compared them with the rates of illness and death. You will find the formulae and charts in Appendix A (page 299).

18. See Beis HaLevi, *Parashas Yisro, Lo sachmod.*
19. *Ohr Yisrael, Sha'arei Yosher*, part 1.

3. EMOTIONAL HEALTH AND PERSONAL DEVELOPMENT

Dietary and lifestyle habits directly affect our emotional well-being, our behavior and even our thought processes. I am not referring here to the negative effects that certain foods have on our moods, nor to the improved emotional outlook that comes with feeling better about yourself. I am referring to what Rambam says:

> Bad habits such as [bad] eating and drinking habits harm one's behavior characteristics (*middos*), while a good regimen greatly improves one's behavior characteristics.[20]

The constitution of the body affects the qualities of the soul. In other words, our physical health affects our emotional health. Since eating habits affect the constitution of the body, it follows that our eating habits also affect our behavior characteristics. This has amazing ramifications for us.

In *Moreh Nevuchim*,[21] Rambam states explicitly:

> The third class of "evils" comprises those which everyone causes himself by his own action…These originate from excessive desire for eating, drinking…indulgence in undue measure or in an improper manner of eating bad food. This brings disease upon the body and soul. The sufferings of the body in this respect are well-known.
>
> [Regarding the soul,]…properties of the soul depend on the condition of the body…[and] the soul, when accustomed to superfluous things, acquires a strong habit of desiring things which

---

20. *Treatise on Asthma* 1:2. See also *Medical Aphorisms* 17:17,18. Rambam's statement was said in the name of Galen. Galen himself devotes a whole section to this subject, called "The Soul's Dependence on the Body." See P.N. Singer, *Galen: Selected Works* (New York: Oxford World's Classics, 1997), pp. 150–176 (the exercise with the small ball).
21. 3:12.

are unnecessary for the preservation of the individual. This desire is without limit.

Rambam's writings are filled with how overindulgence in food and drink damage a person's behavior characteristics.[22] He compares this type of person to an animal,[23] who strengthens his animal instinct and weakens his intellect.[24] Sa'adia Gaon also writes that overindulgence in food dulls the mind and changes a person's disposition, inclining him to greediness and gluttony. The result is that "he comes to resemble the dogs."[25]

Our eating habits also affect our character traits that are not associated with eating. Here is how this occurs.

In Chapter 2, I discussed how habits mold the subconscious mind and touch on some of the deepest aspects of our inner beings. We all know that our physical muscles need to be exercised or else they atrophy. The same applies to our emotional muscles, for which the Subconscious Accumulation Process is responsible. When we exercise them they become stronger, and when we neglect them they weaken – quickly.[26]

Look at it this way. If a person succumbs to an unhealthy craving, he is flexing and empowering his negative emotional muscles and the probability of succumbing again to an unhealthy craving is increased. But if

---

22. *Shemoneh Perakim*, Chapter 4; *Moreh Nevuchim* 3:8, 3:35,38.
23. *Shemoneh Perakim*, Chapter 5; *Regimen of Health* 1:3.
24. See *Chovos HaLevavos, Sha'ar Avodas HaElokim*, Chapter 5, where the "intellect" warns the "soul" (*nefesh*) of excess eating and drinking because it is one of the main roots of contemptible behavior characteristics. See also *Chovos HaLevavos, Sha'ar Yichud HaMa'aseh*, Chapter 5, which warns that overindulgence even in permitted eating and drinking habits can lead to indulging in forbidden pleasures. See also *Mishneh Torah, Hilchos De'os* 1:4, where Rambam discusses the "Golden Mean." Quoting *Mishlei* 13:25, he describes the balanced person as wanting only that which the body needs and cannot exist without. See *Sha'arei Teshuvah*, Gate 1:30, which reiterates all these concepts.
25. *Emunos v'De'os*, Ideal Human Conduct, Chapter 5.
26. See *Sifsei Chaim, Middos v'Avodas Hashem*, Anger 1.

he overcomes an unhealthy craving, he builds stronger "emotional muscles" to help him overcome unhealthy cravings in the future.

How does this impact on our behavior characteristics in general? When we work to strengthen a specific "emotional muscle," it spills over and affects all our emotions and behavioral characteristics – even those that may not be related to food! As Avraham ben HaRambam tells us, all our behavior characteristics are interconnected.[27] Many people have seen this inner change clearly after internalizing our positive eating habits.

4. SPIRITUAL DEVELOPMENT

Rambam begins his famous chapter on health with the ultimate reason for achieving optimum health:

> A healthy and complete body is among the ways of God because it is impossible to understand or have any knowledge of the Creator when one is sick. Therefore, one must avoid those things which are harmful to the body and habituate oneself to those things which are healthy and strengthen the body.[28]

Similarly, in the Introduction to his *Peirush HaMishnayos*, Rambam writes:

> Rabbi Yehudah HaNasi began the Mishnah with *Seder Zera'im* because it deals with the laws that are specific to agriculture, which is the sustenance of all life. Without food, a person cannot live and serve God in any way. Therefore, he opened with the laws dealing with agriculture.

27. *HaMaspik l'Ovdei Hashem*, Chapter 2, s.v. *al odos*. See also *Madreigas HaAdam, Berur HaMiddos*, Chapters 4 and 5.
28. See *Mishneh Torah, Hilchos De'os* 4:1 and *Shemoneh Perakim*, Chapter 5.

In *Moreh Nevuchim*, his main philosophical work, Rambam writes:

> One of life's goals is to be healthy – in the very best bodily state – because it is impossible for a person to take advantage of his intellectual abilities when he is in pain or sick.[29]

Perhaps this is another reason why Rambam places his health advice in his *Hilchos De'os*, the very same section in which he discusses emotional development and personal improvement. After all, optimum health is a *prerequisite* to the attainment of these goals.

This is how *Chovos HaLevavos*, one of the greatest ethical works ever written, puts it:[30]

> Both your body and soul need care. You strengthen your soul by training it though ethics and wisdom.... You strengthen your body by providing it with nutritious foods and drinks....
>
> If you attend to the body alone, you neglect the purpose of your soul. If you focus on the soul alone, you neglect the needs of your body.... Don't neglect your body's necessities, overwork or weaken it because this will lead to the weakening of both your body and soul.

In general, guarding your health, which includes permanent weight loss, is included in the verse, "You shall be very careful for your souls."[31]

True spirituality is about perfecting simple, everyday acts. I know this may seem much less exciting but it is the truth. As Rambam writes:

> One should direct all of his activities regarding physical health and personal existence so that his limbs serve as the perfect media for

29. See *Moreh Nevuchim* 3:27.
30. *Chovos HaLevavos, Sha'ar Cheshbon HaNefesh* 3:25.
31. *Devarim* 4:15; see *Kitzur Shulchan Aruch* 32.

the powers of the soul. This way your soul will be able to perform ethical and intellectual activities without interference.... This level of conduct is very elevated and hard to attain. Only a few will attain it, and only after much habituation. When the [entire] existence of a person is directed toward this end, I say that he is no less than the prophets....

Regarding this it is written, "And you shall love God, your Lord, with all your heart and with all your soul" [*Devarim* 6:5] – i.e. direct all the elements of your soul to one purpose, which is to love God.

Similarly, King Solomon said in his wisdom, "Know Him in all your ways" [*Mishlei* 3:6].... [32]

In this way, one will be serving God constantly. [33]

Ultimately, all the incentives in the world are useless unless we ask the following question: Do we really want to lose weight and gain health? *That is the question.* Saying Yes but then continuing with our old habits, even if we modify them slightly, cannot work. But if the answer is honestly Yes, then let's do what *will* work – it will transform our lives!

As I pointed out in the Introduction, it is truly amazing that improving our eating and lifestyle habits is a gateway to achieving all that these wonderful (and necessary) incentives promise. Why wait until illness forces us to make the correct choices?

I don't know about you, but I would rather make the right choices *now* – and be healthy and vibrant – than be forced to make the same changes under duress, from the doctor's office or a hospital bed!

32. See *Shemoneh Perakim*, Chapter 5. A similar, shortened version of this passage is found in *Mishneh Torah, Hilchos De'os* 3:2,3.
33. See *Mishneh Torah, Hilchos De'os* 3:3.

IN SUMMARY

There are four main incentives for making a change in our eating and lifestyle habits:

1. External appearance

2. Optimum health and disease prevention

3. Emotional health and personal development

4. Spiritual development

Contemplating our different incentives can have a very powerful effect on our perception, attitude and behavior. They play a very important part in the process of breaking entrenched bad habits.[34]

Whenever possible, review your incentives in your mind or out loud. You could even write them down and tack them onto places where you can see them during the day.

---

34. We all know that breaking bad habits can be difficult. *Chovos HaLevavos* (*Sha'ar Avodas HaElokim*, Chapter 5) writes that it will be easier when you weigh the benefits against the negative consequences you suffer by continuing with them. Some general incentives have been added to our practical program of Contemplation. See Chapter 12 of this book.

INSIGHTS AND SUCCESS STORIES

Sarah from United States lost 20 pounds – emotional growth

To be honest, my main incentive for going on the Life-Transforming Diet was to lose weight. I suppose the health aspect also played a small role. But I did not know about the emotional and psychological benefits of the diet. Since I have been on this program I have seen a major change in my general mood and emotional reactions. I am much more patient and much less impulsive.

Leah from South Africa's Poem

I find that repeating this poem helps me remember my incentives when I need to. It strengthens my "muscle of resolve" to make the correct choices:

I want to be **healthy**
emotionally wealthy
And thereby **prevent disease**.

I want to feel light
Like a bird in flight
And I want to feel at ease.

I aim to **look good**
Both inside and out
To become more stable
In tune and devout.

I am **creative**
That means I can choose
To develop my habits –
And my impulses defuse.

CHAPTER 5
TRANSFORMING AT
THE RIGHT PACE

ANIMAL VERSUS HUMAN

Habit formation is not a phenomenon unique to man. Past experiences of animals also have an impact on them. Accumulation of impressions made on an animal's memory will eventually cause it to make "conscious" decisions. For example, a dog will change its direction and run toward a person who is playful, whereas it will run away from someone who angrily raises a stick against him. So what is the difference between the human mind and the animal "mind"?

An animal is only *reactive*, whereas a human being *can also choose to be creative*.

While it seems that animals "think," the progression of their "thoughts" is limited to reaction to external stimuli as well as immediate self-gratification and avoidance of pain or danger.[1] Natural instincts or trained reactions determine an animal's every response. When faced with two opposing feelings simultaneously, the strongest feeling at that moment always prevails. An animal cannot calculate future consequences!

This "reactive mind" also factors very prominently in human beings, most notably when we are asleep. As Rambam writes, while dreaming, different

---

1.   See *Cheshbon HaNefesh* 2 and 96.

thoughts revolve in our minds[2] and we can only *react* to them; there is no possibility of "creative" intervention. That is why we experience a confused collection of images and memories in our dreams.

When we are awake, our "reactive mode" is just as active but now it runs in the background. This is the Subconscious Accumulation Process, which was discussed in detail in Chapter 2. The major difference is that when we are conscious, we can also be *creative*. Our intellect has the ability to create and impose order because it is not dependent on external stimuli. It can direct the Subconscious Accumulation Process. We can choose how we will respond to any situation or experience instead of simply being a slave to our instinctive reactions. It is our intellect and power of discernment which makes us unique from the rest of creation.[3] This is the essence of man.[4]

Thus, a dynamic relationship is set in motion between instincts (i.e. the "reactive mind") and intellect (i.e. the "creative mind"). The potential clash or harmony between these two modes affects almost every decision we make.[5] The "creative mind" has to learn to work with its partner, the "reactive mind." But whenever the intellect is not exerting its influence then our thought process functions in much the same manner as that of an animal's – our reactive mode is dominant. [6]

This dynamic between creative and reactive responses plays itself out many times a day in our food habits. We can choose to initiate the creative process so that positive eating and lifestyle habits become second nature.

2. See *Shemoneh Perakim*, Chapter 2.
3. *Chovos HaLevavos, Sha'ar HaBechinah*, Chapter 5.
4. *Moreh Nevuchim* 1:1.
5. Our Sages referred to the intellect as the *yetzer ha-tov* (good inclination) and our base instincts as the *yetzer ha-ra* (evil inclination). See *Ohr Yisrael*, Letter 30, and *Chovos HaLevavos, Sha'ar HaAvodah*, concerning the debate between intellect and spirit (*nefesh*).
6. *Cheshbon HaNefesh* 97, footnote.

Alternatively, we can shortsightedly choose to react and continue giving in to all of our cravings, allowing bad habits to take control. [7]

WHAT IS THE RIGHT PACE?

When training an animal, a smart master strikes a balance between discipline and caretaking. He knows that if he overburdens the animal and restricts its provisions, the animal's health will be compromised and eventually it will try to attack him. On the other hand, if he pampers the animal, it will become lazy and eventually subjugate its master to fulfill its every whim. A delicate balance is required to condition and train the animal.[8]

The intellect provides us with the ability to control our "animal spirit" – the reactive mind. But like training an animal, real and permanent change requires a delicate balance between making outer changes and making inner changes. If change is too rapid, it will derail the Subconscious Accumulation Process.[9] Therefore, if we really want to change then we have to move at the right pace.[10]

Sadly, extreme, unnatural and "fad" diets are very popular. They pander to the illusive dream of the overweight person for an instant miracle solution that will cause excess weight to just disappear. Yet statistics show that extreme diets and radical initial phases of diets usually end in

7. See also *Ohr Yisrael, Sha'arei Ohr*, Chapter 1.
8. *Cheshbon HaNefesh*, Introduction, point 4.
9. This is a main theme in *Cheshbon HaNefesh*. See the Introduction there, as well as points 16, 17, 21, 60 and 62.
10. "Constant character improvement is overwhelming. One should seek council on how to strike a balance." *Ohr Yisrael*, Letter 30.

disappointment. You simply cannot fight human nature and its established habits for too long!

The following analogy illustrates this point further. It seems amazing that a bodybuilder can pick up very heavy weights. However, the bodybuilder has conditioned himself step by step over time. Beginning with lighter weights, he has built his muscles up until they are able to lift extraordinarily heavy weights.[11] Had he pushed himself too hard along the way, he could have injured himself. On the other hand, if he had been too lax, he would have seen no results. In order to see optimum results, he had to strike a balance between the two.

Similarly, if we really want to succeed in gaining health and losing weight, then we have to move at the right pace. This is the only way to unleash the power of the Subconscious Accumulation Process.

There are other reasons why extreme or haphazard measures are bound to fail in the long term. For one, an extreme program is devastating to both the physical and the emotional health of the body. As Rambam writes:

> One's usual custom and habit is fundamental for maintaining health.... One should not change his habits all at once, in eating, drinking or exercise.... Changing one's habit all at once results in illness.[12]

> It is impossible to go suddenly from one extreme to the other. Therefore, it is not possible according to the nature of man

---

11. See *Cheshbon HaNefesh*, point 21: "The story is told of a Greek wrestler who would carry a calf on his shoulders for a few hours a day. He continued doing this until the calf was three years old. Although the calf grew heavier, he was still able to lift it. People who watched him were amazed by his strength. Those who did not witness him personally, did not believe what they heard about his strength. None of them realized that he had simply conditioned his body over time."
12. *Regimen of Health* 4:15.

> to suddenly discontinue everything to which he has been
> habituated.... human nature always likes that to which it is
> habituated.[13]

Furthermore, we have already seen how habits become second nature and transform the very root of the subconscious mind. So making a drastic change in them is much the same as suddenly switching from hot water to cold water in a shower!

Bad eating habits also differ from other bad habits such as smoking and alcohol consumption because it is impossible to go "cold turkey" from food. We encounter food much of the day, as we need it in order to survive. There is no way to simply give it up! So we constantly have to contend with a steady array of enticing foods and established bad eating habits.

For all these reasons, sudden or extreme measures do not work with food and eating habits in the long run. And that is why it is crucial not to jump stages in this program.

I know that it is often very hard to contain the excitement and determination when beginning a new eating regime. After all, we want to succeed! And we want to succeed *now* – especially if we've "done it all before." So our natural temptation is to skip stages in order to try and speed up the process.

However, it is vital not to jump the gun! It is crucial to stick to the Phases as they are outlined in this book. Each stage has been specifically designed from a physical and psychological perspective. I will explain everything in detail as we go along. Don't worry; the Life-Transforming Diet is geared so that it will not be long before you can customize and adapt its principles to your particular routine and preferences.

---

13. *Moreh Nevuchim* 3:32.

FORMING NEW HABITS

In accordance with Rambam's caution, ours is a system of gradual behavior modification and habit formation. We introduce one positive habit each week. Thus, the first week you will make only one change. The second week, you will make only one change and continue with the change you made in the first week. The third week, you will make only one change and continue with the changes you made in the previous weeks, and so on.

It is important to make only the one change of the new week. The rest of your schedule should stay exactly the same. The program will guide you step by step, and will tell you exactly what to do.

Some people who have tried the Life-Transforming Diet say that they feel hypocritical because they don't feel like they're "on a diet." Others go to the opposite extreme and think, "I've started the diet, so I can overindulge the rest of the day." I say, just follow the clear guidelines. The rest of the time, continue as before. This means, do not add extra restrictions or extra indulgences. Eat normally and concentrate on our positive changes. The point is that we are changing one thing at a time so that the changes will remain permanent. Very soon, your progress will be rapid if you follow the instructions. It will happen at the right pace *for you*.

I suggest that you read the section on perceptions in Chapter 12 as well as re-read the section on habit formation in Chapter 2, so that you are clear about what we are doing and what we are trying to achieve.

DISTORTION AND REALITY

There is another reason why it is crucial to stick to the order and content of the Phases exactly as they are outlined throughout this book.

I have found that many overweight people harbor preconceived notions about what constitutes "successful dieting." They believe that they need diet shakes, calorie counting, food group restrictions or general food restrictions in order to lose weight. The worst part is that because of these preconceived notions, the basic principles of our program often become distorted. Granted this is done unconsciously, but what amazes me is that there are those who continue with their old habits and yet genuinely believe that they are following the Life-Transforming Diet – by the book!

I repeat, ours is not a system of deprivation or restriction, and I urge you not to be afraid to wholeheartedly trust that you *will* lose weight and gain health if you follow our guidelines. You will enjoy the freedom of not limiting yourself beyond the dictates of the Phases. But please don't look simultaneously for old methods of dieting – we know that they don't work in the long run.

For example, on this system, you should never feel hungry! If you do, then you are probably unconsciously distorting a principle and adding restrictions onto yourself that are not prescribed by the dictates of the Phases.

We will teach you how to eat the right foods at the right time. We will also teach you how to continue positively if you slip at any stage, without resorting to old crash diet methods. We will teach you how to gradually change your established habits for new, healthy, balanced and slimming habits which will enable you to be normal weight – while looking and feeling healthy.

Thus, if you continue to count calories, skip or skimp at meals, or drink substitute shakes, then be aware that you are not actually following the guidelines of our system. This means that you cannot be reaping the full benefits of this tried and tested way of life. In order to succeed on the Life-Transforming Diet for the long term, please honestly open up your mind: trust the Rambam – trust the system – to help you methodically stick to the Phases' guidelines, which are clearly outlined in the book. You will learn how to eat in any circumstance. The Life-Transforming Diet is about changing our relationship with food and liberating ourselves from the idea that losing weight involves some type of suffering.

CLOTHES

If your intention is to lose weight, I suggest that you begin now by getting rid of all your clothes that are bigger than your current size. *You are never going to wear them again.* The Life-Transforming Diet is so practical and effective that there is no reason in the world why those larger clothes should have any place in your closet (or in your mind). By now it should be clear that this is not a fad, extreme or short-term crash diet that will ultimately disappoint you.

As you start losing weight, get your clothes adjusted to your smaller size as soon as possible. Buying some new clothes along the way can also act as a wonderful incentive for maintaining your progress. It is an exhilarating feeling when you start to drop in clothes sizes. You will never need to move up a size again. Most likely you will find yourself playing "catch up" with your rapid drop in sizes.

Our clothes are a better gauge of weight loss than any bathroom scale! In fact, the scale has caused many a dieter to abandon his or her efforts to lose weight – or at the very least, to become demoralized. Therefore, *never weigh yourself more than once a week*. In fact, it is a good idea to take the scale out of the bathroom so you will not to be tempted to use it more frequently. And when you do weigh yourself, the best time is either Sunday or Friday morning, before you get dressed and before you eat anything.

LOSING WEIGHT CYCLES

In general, there are no set rules of how your body will react to weight loss. Losing weight usually occurs in cycles. It is normal to reach a plateau after losing a significant amount of weight. For instance, after losing twenty to thirty pounds, many people find that they simply stop losing weight. It is as though the body is getting used to its new form. If this happens to you, please be patient and take your eyes off the scale. Don't give the scale the power to make or break you. Soon a new wave of weight loss will begin.

Weight loss patterns are also different after childbirth. A new mother needs time to recuperate, while adjusting to the physical and emotional demands of nursing and nurturing a baby. So, for at least the first three to six months after childbirth, most women experience a much slower pace of weight loss.

The worst thing for a new mother to do at this stage is starve herself. The body needs more energy than usual, especially if the mother is nursing. The new baby literally feeds off the mother's nutrients. The best thing to do is to stick to the guidelines of the Life-Transforming Diet. Most important, the mother of a newborn child should never skimp on food at all. Eating within the guidelines of the system will leave her feeling satisfied while her body is recuperating.

It is time to turn those frightening health statistics around!

Though you may still feel some resistance to change, just try to visualize yourself looking and feeling the best you have in years. Moreover, remember that much of our daily routine, to which we cling with loyalty, is habit-based. Some of these habits are the products of indoctrination by the media and the so-called "experts." In many cases, we have neglected simple, time-tested principles that were recorded and proven centuries ago.

So let's begin to "de-indoctrinate" ourselves and return to a way of life that can be truly beneficial. It will not be long before you wonder how you ever lived differently!

THE WEEKEND TRAP

There is certainly no shortage of challenging times when it comes to weight loss. Vacation time and big meal gatherings are familiar examples. But the biggest challenge is probably the weekend – specifically, Shabbos. After all, there is so much unstructured free time and large meals are often the norm. It is a real shame to throw away all the effort we make during the week.

Over the weekend, just one deviation can become two and then three or even more. The next week begins full of sound resolve to get back on track, keeping to the guidelines of the Phases. But every week there is the inevitable weekend trap and we may overdo it again.

Putting on two to three pounds over the weekend will mean having to re-lose them during the next week. This could mean being stuck at the same weight for weeks. So the cycle continues. (A well-known nutritionist finds this syndrome exasperating. "Everything is thrown away when the Shabbos meals come around!" she says.)

Interestingly, this pattern is less problematic while maintaining our correct weight. Nonetheless, it is risky to deviate on weekends as a rule because the Subconscious Accumulation Process, fueled over the weekends, could eventually overwhelm our good eating habits during the rest of the week. While losing weight, this pattern clearly can stall weight loss.

If we perceive the Shabbos meals to be just too hard to handle, we set ourselves up for failure. Have a little "chat" with yourself. It will encourage your psyche to focus on safeguarding the past week's successes by continuing your good habits right through Shabbos. Of course Shabbos meals can be challenging, but they are also an opportunity to display your newly acquired, positive eating habits. Focus on your long-term goal of optimum health and weight loss.

We will clearly outline how to cope with the challenges of extra food over Shabbos and at big meal gatherings so that you can really enjoy your meals and come away without regrets. I will discuss all the meals on Shabbos as they become applicable at the different stages of our system.

Remember: The Life-Transforming Diet allows us to live our lives to the full. By planning ahead and remaining calm, we are able to completely participate in all of life's occasions.

THE PHASES

There are **3 Phases** in the Life-Transforming Diet. While the Phases themselves are original, their underlying method and implementation is based on Rambam's guidelines and a personal development approach[14] which aims to break entrenched habits, redesign new positive ones and assist the Subconscious Accumulation Process.

3 PHASES
Phase 1 – The Foundation Phase
Phase 2 – The Accumulation Phase
Phase 3 – The Integration Phase
Goal Weight

---

14. This is based on the system of self-improvement outlined in *Cheshbon HaNefesh*.

We will begin each Phase with a short description of its purpose. Then we will describe each week of the Phase, beginning with the theory and ending off with the Practical Method, which summarizes the day-to-day implementation for that week.

INSIGHTS AND SUCCESS STORIES

Ita from South Africa – weight gain medication

I am on medication which was causing me to gain weight. Fearing that it was impossible for me to lose weight, I felt defeated before I began. After reading about building positive habits through Accumulation of Traces, however, I realized that this system is not an all-or-nothing affair. I made one dietary change and one small daily addition to my (non-existent) exercise schedule and decided to take it day by day. Each day would create one more "trace impression."

I noticed a weight change in the right direction. This meant that the tide had finally turned. Now that I have experienced that I can stick to a plan and that it is possible for me to lose weight again, I will hopefully have the motivation to persevere on the Life-Transforming Diet. Thank you.

Tehilla from England – I want to do it "by the book"

I have to admit that originally I began the Life-Transforming Diet by cherry-picking the stages in order to try and speed things up. You see, I am definitely a non-conformist at heart and so I did it my way. I lost thirteen pounds very quickly – without waiting to implement the changes gradually the way the book suggests. I was ecstatic.

But then I started putting the pounds back on because my new habits were not firmly established. I know that I always like a good shortcut – but shortcuts often seem to take the long way around in the end! Now I just want to start the Life-Transforming Diet all over again – right from the beginning – to do it exactly by the book this time. I have come to really appreciate this well-thought-out program.

CHAPTER 6
PHASE 1

PHASE 1 AT A GLANCE

Week 1 High-Water-Content (HWC) Meal once a day

Week 2 Five to ten minutes of cardiovascular exercise five times a
week

Week 3 Substitution Method between meals

Week 4 Main One-Concentrated-Food (CF) Meal once a day

Week 5 Light One-Concentrated-Food (CF) Meal once a day

THE FOUNDATION PHASE

Building a house begins with the *foundation stage*. This stage can take quite
some time, during which everything looks like a mess to the untrained eye.
The walls have not yet been built and the layout of the bedrooms cannot
be seen. However, professionals know that this is the most important stage.
For them, everything is clear.

Conceptually, we can all appreciate that the foundation stage is absolutely
necessary. After all, without a solid foundation, the building will fall down.
So even though the final construction stages as well as furnishing the
building are often more exciting, there is no way to take a shortcut. The
foundation must be set in place.

Building a foundation applies to creating any lasting structures in life,
whether physical, spiritual or emotional. It is most certainly true about
losing weight. In my opinion, ignoring this stage is one of the main
reasons why so many diets fail in the long term. This program also could
have started with a "big bang." However, an initial impetus of dramatic,
simultaneous changes cannot be sustained in the long term because a

solid foundation of change was not established. Initial weight loss and excitement start to dissipate quickly. *This downslide has nothing to do with our ability or inability to lose weight, and is certainly not the result of lack of willpower.* Quite simply, without a very solid foundation, it is only a matter of time before any structure falls, leaving more of a mess and greater damage than there was in the beginning.

What is the use of short-term, superficial results? We know from the Rambam that our minds and bodies are not ready for drastic change – and we have all seen it time and again in different aspects of our lives!

Therefore, Phase 1 begins with setting firm foundations in place. Each principle is implemented at a steady pace, so do not leave out anything, and please resist the temptation to jump stages! I know that past perceptions together with established diet expectations militate against accepting these new dieting priorities. Many start the Life-Transforming Diet thinking that they will jump ahead and gain the benefits of weight loss before the appropriate time, only to realize that they need to start again and follow the guidelines exactly – even though this may not initially feel right. I repeat, make only the one change of the new week. The rest of your schedule should stay exactly the same. Do not add extra restrictions or extra indulgences. Eat normally and concentrate on your positive changes. The point is that we are changing one thing at a time so that our changes will remain permanent.

In the first four weeks, some people lose a little weight, some lose a lot of weight and others remain constant. It does not matter, because *weight loss is not the focus during the first four to five weeks*. Don't feel disheartened; we are looking at enduring weight loss which continues until your goal weight! This might not make sense within the accepted diet mentality – but the accepted mentality does not produce lasting results. Our aim right now is behavior modification; in other words, changing our well-established habits.

I suggest that you give yourself the allotted time of Phase 1 – five weeks – to establish healthy habits before you start weighing yourself. Weigh yourself in the beginning, just so you have a record. Then take the scale out of your bathroom and free yourself from its bondage for a month!

Others have embarked on this program and you can too. I assure you that you are laying down a solid basis for future *permanent* results.

PHASE I

In terms of our primary principles, i.e. food quantity and exercise, this is what you can expect in Phase 1:

Week 1: Food quantity

In the first week, we focus on how many meals a day we should eat.

Week 2: Exercise

In the second week, we begin to implement a basic, well-balanced exercise program.

Week 3: Food quantity

In the third week, we focus on eating between meals.

Weeks 4 and 5: Food quantity

During these weeks, we will focus on food quantity at the meals.

PHASE 1 / WEEK 1

Method   High-Water-Content (HWC) Meal once a day

HOW MANY MEALS

We have learned that when it comes to diet, our primary concern must be food quantity. I mentioned that there are three different ways you can overeat: at a meal, between meals, and by having too many meals.

Let's begin with "having too many meals."

It is clear from the Talmud,[1] Rambam, *Shulchan Aruch*[2] and later authorities[3] that the average healthy person did not eat more than two main meals a day.

Rambam writes that the number of meals eaten per day is of primary importance for maintaining health.[4] Moreover, he says:

> People have different habits regarding when they eat. Most of them eat in the morning and evening....
>
> The general rule to rely on is that strong people can eat what they need at one meal [per day]. But it is a grave mistake for weak people, such as the elderly and convalescents, to have all their nourishment at one meal. Instead, their food should be divided

---

1. *Pesachim* 12b; *Shabbos* 10a.
2. *Orach Chaim* 157.
3. *Kitzur Shulchan Aruch* 32:10. .
4. See *Medical Aphorisms* 17:19.

in proportion to their strength, eating small quantities at short intervals[5] so that their strength does not fade.[6]

Rambam himself ate one *main* meal a day:

Know that it may happen to someone who eats only once a day that by the evening his stomach is empty.... [7]

I have confirmed from personal experience that if I eat bread [in the evening], even a small amount, I am harmed and my digestion is impaired because of the change in my habit.... I have found that the best thing to do is to eat light tasty foods which are easy to digest. Sometimes I drink soup made from young roosters and then go to sleep...sometimes I eat some pistachio nuts and seedless raisins or raisins and almonds with *fanid*[8].... During the winter, I take a glass of wine when it is cold. In general, one should not spend the night in a hungry state...[9]

It is clear from the Rambam that a healthy person should not be eating more than two main meals a day. Furthermore, eating frequent smaller meals a day is suggested only for weaker people such as the elderly or a recovering patient.

Most of us think we need at least three large meals a day to maintain a healthy body, and as a result we clog up and overburden our digestive systems. Then we wonder why we suffer from depleted energy levels, weight problems and frequent illness!

5. Elsewhere, Rambam writes that the elderly should eat small amounts of food three times a day. See *Medical Aphorisms* 17:29 and 20:8.
6. *Treatise on Asthma* 6:1.
7. Ibid.
8. See ibid., 6:4, Gerrit Bos translation (Provo, UT: Brigham Young University Press, 2002).
9. *Treatise on Asthma* 6:4.

We could accustom ourselves to eating only two meals a day, but we live in a world where three meals a day is the accepted norm. So how can we eat three meals a day without it ruining the balance of our two main meals?

THE HIGH-WATER-CONTENT MEAL SOLUTION

Here is a solution: One meal a day should consist mainly of high-water-content foods. These are fruits and vegetables. (Any other foods are considered concentrated foods.)

The National Cancer Institute (NCI) states that fruits and vegetables should be the foundation of a healthy diet, and recommends that we eat five to nine servings every day. Fruits and vegetables are high in nutrients and fiber and low in calories. If you eat more fruits and vegetables and fewer high-calorie foods, and you will find it much easier to control your weight. Moreover, a growing body of research proves that fruits and vegetables are critical to promoting good health. In addition to fiber, they are packed with essential vitamins, minerals and disease-fighting phytochemicals. Eating plenty of fruits and vegetables every day can help reduce your risk of heart disease, high blood pressure, type 2 diabetes and certain cancers.

A majority fruit or vegetable meal is the perfect solution for our third, "non-main meal." Because a fruit or vegetable meal is easy to digest and low in calories, it will not overburden our digestive systems. Instead, it will provide us with increased energy levels, improved health and a jump start to weight loss. Furthermore, this highly nutritious meal is a great way to help meet the NCI's suggested dietary guidelines.

It appears from Rambam's writings that a high-water-content meal will not ruin the balance of meals, as Rambam lists only protein and starches as "main foods."[10] Thus, the fruit or vegetable meal is not considered a "main meal." You are still eating three meals a day, but they are technically two meals a day according to Rambam's requirements.

I call this meal the high-water-content (HWC) meal because fruits and vegetables are the only foods with a very high water content. Besides carrying nutrients into the body, the water contained in fruits and vegetables performs the essential function of cleansing and detoxifying the body of wastes.[11]

Rambam suggested that "tree" fruit should not be eaten in quantity, but said that fresh or dried figs, grapes and almonds were always beneficial although not to be eaten "constantly."[12] He also advocated the consumption of olives and raisins.[13] He wrote that eating melon in the morning on an empty stomach is very beneficial.[14]

We must keep in mind that in Rambam's day there was rapid spoilage of fresh fruit. As there was no refrigeration or efficient means of transport, by the time the fresh fruit reached the marketplace or homes, it had been exposed to a long, hot journey on the back of a donkey or camel, sometimes under the scorching sun of the desert. Thus, this might be the reason Rambam proposed limiting the quantity of fresh fruit consumed and advocated the consumption of dried and cured fruit.

Rambam also states explicitly that people should not be surprised that eating fruit does not result in adverse effects because different cultures, climates and predispositions cause us to react differently to specific foods.[15]

---

10. *Regimen of Health* 1:6.
11. See Harvey and Marilyn Diamond, *Fit for Life* (London: Bantam Books, 1987), p. 36.
12. *Mishneh Torah, Hilchos De'os* 4:11; see also *Regimen of Health* 1:12.
13. See *Medical Aphorisms* 20:56,57.
14. See *Regimen of Health* 1:11.
15. *Regimen of Health* 1:13.

Furthermore, Rambam's writings are filled with guidelines on how and when to eat fruit.

For these reasons, in addition to the fact that most nutritionists and doctors consider fruit to be an essential part of our diet, we advocate the eating of fruits at the correct times. However, if you are not satisfied with our reasoning, it is certainly still possible to follow all the guidelines of the Phases without eating too much fruit – or even without eating fruit at all. For example, your High-Water-Content Meal could be a vegetable meal such as a vegetable soup and large platter of fresh salad with salad dressing. And between meals, there are certainly enough choices other than fruit (see Phase 1, Week 3). In the Life-Transforming Diet, there are so many ways to customize your own personal program within its flexible guidelines.

YOUR PERSONAL HWC MEAL CHOICES

Fruit HWC Meal

–   Make sure you are eating enough fruit[16] or salad. The fruit should fill a cereal bowl – at least.

–   Experiment with the different fruit. Some fruits are more filling than others. I like to eat melon in the morning, switching between the different types of melons each day. I also enjoy grapefruit or pomelo.

–   If you want to eat more than one type of fruit at this meal, try combining them. Some people like to mix pineapple with apple, apple with orange, or blueberries with strawberries. There are so many different possible combinations. Regarding melon, many nutritional

16. Be careful not to eat unripe fruits. Rambam writes, "Unripe fruit is like swords to the body" (*Mishneh Torah, Hilchos De'os* 4:11).

experts maintain that it should be eaten alone. Rambam also mentions eating melon *alone in the morning.*[17]

- If, *after sincerely trying,* you find that a fruit meal alone is not filling enough, you may eat the fruit together with a topping of *nuts* (not seeds). Rambam was most fond of almonds and pistachios.[18] Remember: these are just a topping, so don't have more than 90 calories' worth of nuts. This is about twenty pistachios or thirteen medium almonds. This will be 1½ to 2 tablespoons (0.5–0.6 oz.) of nuts. (For amounts of other nuts, see Chapter 13.) If you feel that once you start eating the nuts you are having a hard time controlling the quantity consumed, it may be a good idea to wait until later on in the Phases before adding them to your diet.

Vegetable HWC Meal

- If you are eating vegetables for your HWC meal, fill a large plate or bowl with salad or vegetables. You can also begin with a vegetable soup.

- You may use non-starchy vegetables such as lettuce, tomato, peppers, spinach, broccoli, cauliflower, celery, asparagus, etc. Add a low-fat or nonfat dressing (no hydrogenated oils), or a homemade dressing using olive oil, lemon juice and herbs.

- You may also eat medium-starchy vegetables such as carrots, beets, butternut squash, pumpkin, winter squash and peas at this meal. Some people like to add them to a salad and others like to bake them and eat them separately with a salad.

17. See *Regimen of Health* 1:11.
18. *Treatise on Asthma* 6:4; *Medical Aphorisms* 20:51,78; *Causes of Symptoms* 21; *Mishneh Torah, Hilchos De'os* 4:11.

- If, *after sincerely trying,* you find that this meal alone is not filling enough, you may add a topping of *seeds* (not nuts) such as sunflower or sesame seeds. As above, it should be limited to 90 Calories (see above for measurements).

- Regarding soup, it should consist *only* of vegetables and water. Using a big variety and large amount of vegetables will create a thick texture. Adding some butternut squash and blending the cooked mixture will make it creamy. Don't forget to add spices and herbs, and you have a delicious, satisfying soup. Zucchini soup is one of my favorites. You can even freeze some for another meal.

You will find a full list of fruit and vegetable choices, as well as general foods and their food groups, at the end of Chapter 13. (Please see page 221 for a third meal option, other than fruit and vegetables: any meal less than 250 calories.)

FRUIT AND THE HWC MEAL

If the idea of having one fruit meal a day seems very revolutionary or extreme to you, you should know that there are millions of people who already do this. I am not talking about people who live in the jungle; I am referring to people who live in Western countries! Naturopaths, for instance, prescribe a fruit meal for breakfast.[19] They maintain that the many benefits of fruit can be obtained only if they are eaten on an empty stomach. For example, Professor Celene Bernstein writes:

> When other foods are eaten together with fruit, which is a quicker to digest food, the fruit is held up in the stomach and starts

---

19. See Mary Ann Shearer, *Perfect Weight* (Cape Town: Ibis Books, 2003), p. 9.

fermenting and putrefying. This creates by-products of bacterial decomposition, such as alcohol, acetic acid and ammonia which are poisonous to the body. These toxic by-products irritate the tissues, and waste the energy the body requires to pass them through the alimentary canal. These poisons eventually end up in the blood stream and manifest in various allergies, gas, acid indigestion, flatulence and heartburn.[20]

Rambam's opinion, which was written over eight hundred years ago, is clear:[21]

- One should eat fruit only on an empty stomach.[22]

- One should never combine fruit with a meal.[23]

Consequently, a fruit HWC meal provides the optimum time to eat fruit.

You may be wondering, "I thought fruit should only be eaten alone. So how can I eat a nut topping with my fruit meal?" Interestingly, nuts are considered botanical fruits. We make the same blessing on nuts as we do on fruit. (The only exception is peanuts; they are a legume.) Furthermore, it is apparent from Rambam's writings that nuts can be eaten with fruits. Rambam groups dried fruits together with nuts:

> Dried fruits such as raisins, dried figs and the kernels of dried almonds and pistachio are not bad.[24]

---

20. Celene Bernstein, *Health Seekers* (Florida, South Africa: Vivlia Publishers, 1998), p. 58.
21. Later we will see that according to Rambam, some fruits can be eaten at least thirty minutes before a meal, and small quantities of constipating fruits can be eaten at the end of a meal.
22. See *Treatise on Asthma* 3:9.
23. See *Regimen of Health* 1:13. See also *Causes of Symptoms* 10–11 and *Mishneh Torah, Hilchos De'os* 4:6.
24. *Regimen of Health* 1:13.

Even more explicitly, he writes:

> Almonds are among the most salutary of fruits and specifically strengthen the stomach and liver.... Dried figs together with nuts or almonds are beneficial. [25]

Regarding vegetables, Rambam does not say that these high-water-content foods can only be eaten alone. Naturopaths maintain this same opinion. I have seen this explanation: "Vegetables do not need their own specific digestive juices. They will break down in either medium, acid or alkaline [digestive juices]."[26] So you can eat vegetables alone or at any meal. But fruit should always be eaten alone.

THE HWC ADVANTAGE

Some people who have never tried eating a high-water-content meal are very skeptical when they first read about it. They immediately think, "A high-water-content meal will never be enough to satisfy me." I ask you to enter this Phase with an open mind. You will probably be very pleased with the results!

First, there is the fiber factor. Some of the best sources of fiber are fruits, vegetables, seeds and nuts. According to Barbara Rolls, Ph.D., author of *The Volumetrics Eating Plan*, fiber can help us eat less and lose weight. Joanne Slavin, Ph.D., an obesity researcher at the University of Minnesota, says dietary fiber makes us feel fuller. Some studies have shown that large amounts of fiber in the diet can help regulate blood glucose and insulin.

25. *Medical Aphorisms* 20:51,78.
26. *Fit For Life*, p. 53.

Perhaps this is the reason why people who eat higher-fiber diets tend to weigh less and are less prone to gain weight as they age.[27]

Secondly, the HWC meal consists of light, tasty foods that are easy to digest. Digesting food properly may be more effective in preventing hunger than eating large amounts of food. It is not unusual to find people who eat very large or frequent meals during the day and still feel hungry most of the time. Since they are not digesting their food properly, they are not absorbing the nutrients from their food efficiently. This can leave the body craving the nutrients it requires.[28] The National Cancer Institute states that fruits and vegetables are a natural source of energy and give the body many nutrients we need to keep going.

Finally, although we will not discuss eating between meals until Phase 1, Week 3, if you get hungry before the next meal, eat some more fruit or vegetables, or try having a hot drink such as hot water, herbal tea or decaffeinated coffee.[29] You certainly do not have to fast between meals. People who have a hot drink early in the morning or at breakfast would be much better delaying this hot drink until early mid-morning. As times passes, you will notice that you will eat less food between meals.

The reality is that the first few days of breaking any bad habit can be hard. This is true about any program of change. The subconscious accumulation of previous habits compels us to continue with our old ways and behaviors. Rambam sums it up perfectly:

> How can you expect a small portion of light and nutritious food to be pleasing if you are accustomed to unhealthy, heavy food?[30]

27. For more information, see the Internet reference for Phase 1, Week 1, in Appendix E (page 324).
28. See also *Perfect Weight*, p. 101.
29. See Phase 1, Week 3, where we discuss drinking and the different types of drink.
30. *Introduction to Perek Chelek.*

In my experience, after about two weeks of eating the HWC meal, most people literally get hooked on it. Any short-term discomfort is the result of an inner shuffle of the subconscious accumulation of traces. Very shortly, you will start to experience a significant inner shift in the direction of your new habit. Remember, this is the only change that you will be making in your first week. It is also the only change you will make to your meal schedule until Week 4 of this Phase.

When should we eat this high-water-content meal? Should it be eaten for breakfast, lunch or dinner?

MEAL FLEXIBILITY

Regarding eating a fruit meal for breakfast, bestselling authors Harvey and Marilyn Diamond write:

> The reasoning behind eating exclusively fruit in the morning is tied closely to the efficient functioning of your body cycles.
>
> In weight loss we are interested in not blocking the elimination cycle.
>
> The elimination cycle takes place from 4:00 A.M. to noon time. Digestion of conventional food takes more energy than any other body process. Fruit demands the least amount of energy for its digestion. So it is most beneficial for fruit to be the only foods consumed during the elimination cycle, if you consume anything at all. Anything else halts the elimination process and the by-products of foods that should have been eliminated are now added to your toxic load and to the unwanted pounds in your body.[31]

31. *Fit for Life*, p. 76.

There are other advantages to having this meal in the morning. First of all, did you know that about 40 percent of Americans skip breakfast altogether? A simple and healthy high-water-content meal for breakfast insures that you do not leave out this important meal. Relative to other nutritious meals – especially cooked meals – this meal is certainly quicker and easier to prepare. Furthermore, as mentioned above, according to Rambam, eating melon alone for breakfast is digested well, stimulates the elimination cycle and cleanses the body.[32] Most high-water-content foods have a similar cleansing effect. It's a great feeling to start the day on a cleansing note! A good beginning predisposes us to a good ending.

I have heard some people say that breakfast is the most important meal of the day and we should be eating a large breakfast. On the Life-Transforming Diet, we believe that breakfast is like any other meal – although, as we explained above, there are good reasons why breakfast should be your lightest meal of the day.

Even in the times of the Talmud, breakfast was not considered one of the main meals. It was not eaten by everyone, and when it was eaten, it consisted of one mouthful of plain bread and some water – more like a snack.[33] An HWC breakfast is a much more filling "extra" meal.

Still, everyone is different and we all have our unique schedules. I believe that flexibility is crucial in any long-term eating and lifestyle plan. Furthermore, our main reason for eating this HWC meal is that it allows us the opportunity to have three meals a day while it is still considered as if we are eating two main meals a day. Therefore, it doesn't matter which

32. See *Regimen of Health* 1:11.
33. See *Sukkah* 26a and Rashi ad loc., s.v. *kedeta'im*. See also Tosafos on *Sukkah* 26a, s.v. *tarti oh tlas*. See also *Tur, Orach Chaim* 155:1; *Mishnah Berurah* 157:5 and *Biur Halachah* ad loc., as well as *Be'er Heitev, Orach Chaim* 155:2.

meal you choose to be your HWC meal. You decide what suits you best. In fact, eating the HWC meal for either lunch or dinner also has advantages.

Some Jewish[34] (and medical) sources feel that making lunch a light meal will give you more energy during the day and will enable you to learn Torah better.

The *Kitzur Shulchan Aruch*[35] writes about eating a light dinner. He lists the benefits:

1. It is more beneficial to the body, and aids in general preservation of health.

2. The quality of sleep will be light and invigorating, allowing you to awaken in the morning at the correct time.

3. Other complications which may be caused by excessive eating can be avoided.

Let me also add that eating a lighter meal for dinner is beneficial for people who suffer from heartburn. Large meals at night, especially close to bedtime, are a major cause of heartburn and indigestion.

As you can see, there are authoritative opinions to support whatever meal you choose to be the high-water-content meal. Ultimately, you will decide which it is to be: breakfast, lunch or dinner. In truth, it may boil down to this: If there is any meal that you often skip, or if any one of your meals is usually at a time which is inconvenient or busy for you, then this is the meal to choose as your HWC Meal.

For some people, in the morning rush a bowl of fruit is a quick and satisfying breakfast. For others, a lunch of fruit or salad in the middle of a

---

34. *Orchos Tzaddikim, Sha'ar HaAhavah; Be'er Heitev, Orach Chaim* 157. See also *Mishnah Berurah* 157:4.
35. 71:2.

hectic day at work can be a very convenient option. Or for dinner, a bowl or two of vegetable soup and/or salad will leave you feeling light and satisfied before going to bed.

No one has the same schedule or preferences, and therefore flexibility is crucial. The best part is that you will gain health benefits no matter when you choose to eat this meal. However, in general, it is best to stick to a specific meal every day as your high-water-content choice, so that a habit can form. This is certainly true during the first two Phases.

On Shabbos, the time of your HWC meal may alter. This will depend on your preference, as well as the laws concerning the three meals on Shabbos and the different opinions concerning them. This will be discussed in detail below and in Appendix D. You can choose to eat this meal in the late morning (with or after Kiddush), in the afternoon (for *seudah shelishis*) or in the evening (for *melaveh malkah*). Some people will choose to skip this meal on Shabbos.

I have seen people who were extremely obese and obsessive about food who got absolutely hooked on this high-water-content meal. If they could try it and love it, so can you! Once you get used to this invigorating and cleansing meal, you will not turn back. This principle alone has the ability to transform the quality of your life!

HWC MEAL ON SHABBOS

Shabbos is a special day to which we all look forward, a day on which there is a special mitzvah to "enjoy" food.[36] Yet our Sages warn that it is not a time to cultivate bad eating habits or to overeat. In fact, the Vilna Gaon

---

36. See the sources in Appendix D (page 315).

writes that the mitzvah to eat on Shabbos can become a back door for the *yetzer ha-ra* to enter in order to encourage overeating.[37] Moreover, overeating jeopardizes the mitzvah of *oneg Shabbos*.[38] It also stalls weight loss and adversely affects your health. It is therefore imperative that we learn how to draw a balance between indulgence and restraint. Following the Life-Transforming Diet guidelines will help you do just that.

You may choose to eat your HWC Meal for *melaveh malkah* (the Saturday night meal) or *seudah shelishis* (the third Shabbos meal). If you are going to eat bread at these meals, it is best to make the meal a vegetable HWC Meal. There is a difference of opinion whether someone overweight or concerned about their weight must eat bread at these two meals. See Appendix D and ask your Rav. If you do eat bread, one thin slice of challah is enough according to all opinions (see page 322).

There is certainly no obligation to make Kiddush and eat before the second Shabbos meal, so some people wait to eat until this midday meal. However, some women may want to eat in the morning. All opinions hold that you can fulfill the daytime Kiddush obligation with a *melo lugmav* plus a *revi'is* of wine or grape juice (see Appendix D or ask your Rav for the exact amount). After this you can eat some cut-up fruit (which would be considered a mid-morning fruit snack as opposed to an HWC Meal). If you feel that you need to eat *mezonos*, you can eat a *kezayis*.[39] If you eat *mezonos*, it is best to eat cut-up vegetables or a salad with it instead of fruit, because fruit should be eaten on an empty stomach.

---

37. Rabbi Avigdor Miller, Tape #744: "Restricting Free Will."
38. *Shulchan Aruch, Orach Chaim* 291:1.
39. It is impossible to generalize a *kezayis* amount. For example, four Saltines (13 grams), four Snackers (13 grams) or six Tam Tams (19 grams) are each a *kezayis*. Three-quarters of one *rugaleh* (14 grams) or half of a large cookie (25 grams) are each a *kezayis*. It is preferable to eat whole wheat for your *mezonos*. For more information, see Rabbi Yisroel Pinchos Bodner, *Halachos of K'zayis* (Jerusalem: Feldheim Publishers, 2001).

It is certainly best to eat fruit or vegetables at this point because you will still be eating three more meals before the end of the day. If slices of fruit or strips of vegetables are not satisfying enough, you can eat more fruit or vegetables, making this "mid-morning snack" closer in quantity to an HWC Meal. You may also add a topping of nuts to the fruit or a topping of seeds to the vegetables.

These Shabbos guidelines are especially important while you are trying to lose weight. When you are close to your goal weight, you may choose to be more liberal. For example, you may want to eat some cholent at a festive Kiddush, but bear in mind that you will be eating lunch in a very short time. Besides the health implications of eating too much, you may jeopardize *oneg Shabbos* at the main meal, which is an obligation. As the *Shulchan Aruch* says, "A wise man plans ahead by not filling his stomach";[40] otherwise, it can result in gross overeating (*achilah gasah*), which is not considered eating.[41]

The other meals on Shabbos will be discussed when we start to deal with the main meals. We have to be careful not to turn the mitzvah of *oneg Shabbos* into an activity that cultivates bad eating habits or *achilah gasah*, or even jeopardizes the very mitzvah itself. There is more than enough room to apply the Life-Transforming Diet principles more liberally on Shabbos and still not compromise your new, positive lifestyle changes. You can enjoy Shabbos – including your obligation to enjoy your food – without discarding all your hard work during the week.

40. *Shulchan Aruch, Orach Chaim* 291:1.
41. *Mishnah Berurah* 291:4.

PHASE 1 / WEEK 1
PRACTICAL METHOD

YOUR FIRST WEEK

A High-Water-Content Meal once a day is the only change you will make.

Many people sigh with relief that they are not expected to make a lot of extreme changes simultaneously at the start of the Life-Transforming Diet. This fact alone distinguishes our system from others.

1. Choose which meal will be your high-water-content meal – breakfast, lunch or dinner. As you saw above, it is beneficial for you no matter which meal you choose it to be.

If you have no real preference, I suggest that you make breakfast your high-water-content meal. This is merely a recommendation based on experience, but you can certainly make your own choice.

Once you choose which meal will be your high-water-content meal, try to stick to that choice for Phase 1 and Phase 2. As mentioned above, this is important because one of the main goals of the Phases is to help mold positive eating habits. After Phase 2, you can change the position of this meal if you want. In general, however, it is always best to stick to the same eating patterns so that a habit can be formed and reinforced.

2. Choose *what* you will eat for this High-Water-Content Meal – fruit or vegetables. Do not stint on quantity. Remember these guidelines:

For the fruit option:

- Experiment with different fruits.

- If you want more than one type of fruit, try eating a combination of different fruits together (melons should be eaten alone).

- You may add a *topping* of nuts such as almonds or pistachios (1.5–2 Tbsp. / 0.5–0.6 oz.).

For the vegetable option:

- Add a variety of vegetables to your salad with an appetizing, low-fat dressing. You can also eat medium-starchy vegetables separately or in the salad. You may want to start the meal with a vegetable soup.

- You may add a topping of seeds such as sesame (1.5–2 Tbsp. / 0.5–0.6 oz.).

INSIGHTS AND SUCCESS STORIES

Joel from United States – High-Water-Content Meal

I lost 5 pounds in the first two weeks of the Life-Transforming Diet. The only eating change I made was the High-Water-Content Meal for breakfast. I originally thought, "Fruit for breakfast will never work for me," but I decided to give it a try nonetheless. All I can say is that I am hooked. Not only do I love to eat my chilled fruit meal in the morning, but I feel full of energy afterwards. Try it and you'll see for yourself!

Dini from Israel – digestive issues

I have always suffered from digestion problems. It was especially unbearable when I was on a diet which allowed almost no carbohydrates, vegetables and fruits.

From the beginning of Phase 1 on the Life-Transforming Diet, I have experienced big changes. I am drinking more water and enjoying eating the fruits and vegetables. The fruit High-Water-Content Meal helps my system run smoothly. I am very grateful.

PHASE 1 / WEEK 2

Method Five to ten minutes of cardiovascular exercise five times a week
Continue High-Water-Content Meal once a day

WEIGHT LOSS AND HEALTH BENEFITS OF EXERCISE

Must we really exercise in order to lose weight? After all, some diets claim that exercise is not necessary, and we all know people who seem to have lost weight without an exercise program! I can't tell you about other diets, but on the Life-Transforming Diet you can definitely lose weight without exercising.

However...let me give you a startling fact: In the United States, more than 60 percent of the population does not do enough exercise, and more than 25 percent are not active at all in their leisure time.[1] Interestingly, more than 60 percent of Americans are overweight, of which more than 25 percent are considered obese. Is it just a coincidence that the percentage of people who are overweight is the same as the percentage of people who do not do enough exercise? What about the fact that the percentage of people who are obese is the same as the percentage of people who do not do any exercise at all?

1.   See United States Department of Health and Human Services (USDHHS), "Physical Activity and Health: A Report of the Surgeon General," 1996. Unless otherwise noted, statistics in this chapter are quoted by the National Center for Chronic Disease Prevention and Health Promotion.

It may be possible to lose weight without exercising, but most dieters don't. Even if they do manage to lose weight, they are usually not able to maintain their weight loss without exercise.

A workout is often mistakenly measured by how many calories are burned in the process. However, your metabolic rate increases both during and after exercise. The effects last up to forty-eight hours after exercising, enabling your body to work much more efficiently. This leads to weight loss even while you are relaxing!

Interestingly, the body often reacts to dieting by slowing down its metabolic rate. This is especially relevant during the middle-age years, when most people experience a slowing metabolism anyway. But the bottom line is that exercise is vital for you regardless of your situation or age, as it helps speed up your metabolic rate.

There is another important reason to exercise while losing weight. When you lose weight without exercising, you may look the same externally as your counterpart who does exercise, but internally you will look worlds apart.

Exercise burns fat!

If you combine diet with exercise, you will lose weight by reducing body fat and not lean muscle. Almost all your weight loss will result from fat reduction! In contrast, when you lose weight without exercising, you lose about 75 percent body fat and about 25 percent lean body mass. And body composition is crucial for good health.

Remember that the bathroom scale does not measure how much body weight is fat and how much is muscle. Therefore, the scale is not the most reliable gauge of your progress. The real enemy is not your weight but a high body fat percentage.

Furthermore, exercise will improve your physical appearance.

Even if you do succeed in losing weight and keeping it off without exercising, there is still the issue of general health. Today, it is accepted that exercise is one of the most important ingredients in any general health program. In fact, studies show the sensational health benefits of regular exercise.

For one, many serious illnesses can be prevented by exercising. The United States Department of Health and Human Services (USDHHS)[2] states that millions of Americans suffer from chronic illnesses which could be prevented or improved through regular physical activity. One study linked sedentary lifestyles to 23 percent of the deaths from major chronic diseases.[3]

Here are just some of the many other health benefits of exercise:[4]

- Exercise strengthens the heart, reducing the risk of heart disease or a second heart attack. Some research indicates that simply walking briskly for three or more hours a week reduces the risk of coronary heart disease by 65 percent.

- Exercise reduces the risk of type 2 diabetes. It may also decrease insulin requirements for people with diabetes.

- Exercise helps reduce triglyceride levels, which are linked to coronary disease in some people.

- Exercise lowers bad (LDL) cholesterol and raises good (HDL) cholesterol.

2. USDHHS, "Physical Activity Fundamental to Preventing Disease," June 20, 2002.
3. S.M. Teuesch, R.B. Rothenberg et al., "Excess Deaths from Nine Chronic Diseases in the United States, 1986." JAMA 264(20):2554–59 (1998). Quoted in "Physical Activity Fundamental to Preventing Disease."
4. For Internet references backing up the facts and statistics cited throughout Phase 1, Week 2, please see Appendix E, page 324.

- Exercise lowers your risk of having a stroke.

- Exercise helps lower blood pressure.

- Exercise decreases the risk of getting certain types of cancers, such as colon cancer and breast cancer.

- Exercise improves circulation, as it oxygenates the blood. You will feel rejuvenated and energized.

- Exercise accelerates bowel movement by stimulating the peristaltic action of the intestines.[5]

- Exercise tones the body, improving bone structure and reducing the risk of osteoporosis, arthritis and back pain.

- Exercise improves sleep quality.

- Scientific research has shown that exercise can slow the physiological aging clock. It also extends your life expectancy.

- Studies have shown that smokers who exercise regularly are more likely to cut down on or stop smoking.

- Many studies have shown that exercise boosts moods and reduces anxiety, depression and stress.

The importance of exercise and its amazing benefits is certainly not a modern scientific breakthrough. Read what Rambam wrote many centuries ago:

> Hippocrates taught that exercise is a cornerstone in the preservation of health and the repulsion of most illnesses. There is nothing that can substitute for exercise in any way.[6]

---

5. See *Health Seekers*, p.10. See also *Regimen of Health* 1:3.
6. See *Regimen of Health* 1:3; *Medical Aphorisms* 17:1, 2.

> Many serious illnesses would be prevented if people would treat themselves as they treat their pets! A person is careful to take his pet for a walk so that it remains healthy and does not become ill. However, we neglect our own bodies, paying no attention to exercise.[7]

> Without exercise, a good diet alone is not sufficient [for the preservation of health] and eventually medical treatment will be needed.[8]

> A person who does not exercise will suffer from pain and depleted energy levels, even if the correct foods are eaten and all the rules of medicine are followed.[9]

Exercise also has an impact on our food choices and eating habits. Rambam tells us, "A person who customarily exercises before meals does not have to be as careful [with his diet]."[10] In other words, exercise prepares the body so that we can be more liberal with our diet. At the same time, it allows the body to digest quantities of food in a more efficient manner. Rambam writes in his *Commentary on Hippocrates' Aphorisms*, "Physical laborers also have more natural heat because they do a lot of physical activity and therefore they can digest larger amounts of food."[11]

Rambam sums it up in one line:

> Exercise repels the damage done by most of man's bad habits.[12]

Thus, the amount of calories you burn during any particular workout is really one very small part of the process. Exercise is not just a luxury for

---

7. *Regimen of Health* 1:3.
8. *Medical Aphorisms* 18:1.
9. See *Mishneh Torah, Hilchos De'os* 4:15.
10. *Medical Aphorisms* 18:1.
11. *Commentary on Hippocrates' Aphorisms* 1:15.
12. See *Regimen of Health* 1:3.

people who have the time. It is a key component in any health or weight loss program. Its accumulative effects improve your health, weight and emotional well-being.

WHO CAN EXERCISE?

Every person, at every age and in any situation, can benefit from an exercise program. My late grandfather could certainly attest to this. He was almost ninety years old when he passed away, and he exercised right until the end of his life. He rode his stationary bike twice a day as well as adhered to a regular exercise regimen.

The particulars of an exercise program will differ for children, average adults, pregnant women, obese adults, elderly people and those with disabilities or a medical problem. Before embarking on an exercise program, please consult your doctor. Certainly, it is imperative to see a doctor if you have any of the symptoms detailed in the footnote below.[13]

13. a) You have a heart condition or you've had a stroke, and your doctor recommended only medically supervised physical activity. b) If during or right after you exercise, you often have pains or pressure in the left or mid-chest area, left neck, shoulder or arm. c) You've developed chest pain or discomfort within the last month. d) You tend to lose consciousness or fall due to dizziness. e) You feel extremely breathless after mild exertion. f) Your doctor recommended that you take medicine for your blood pressure, a heart condition or a stroke. g) Your doctor said you have bone, joint or muscle problems that could be exacerbated by the proposed physical activity. h) You have a medical condition or other physical reason, not mentioned here, that might need special attention in an exercise program (for example, insulin-dependent diabetes). i) You're middle-aged or older, haven't been physically active, and plan a relatively vigorous exercise program.
    After consulting your doctor, you can start on a gradual, sensible program of increased activity tailored to your needs. (This list was developed from several sources, particularly "The Physical Activity Readiness Questionnaire," British Columbia Ministry of Health, Department of National Health and Welfare, Canada, 1992 [revised].) See first Internet reference for Phase 1, Week 2, on page 324.

No matter what your situation or age, the key to long-term success is to start off small and build up to a moderate, practical and consistent program of exercise. We will soon learn how to do this in a realistic way. In a relatively short time, you will find that you are fitter than most people who are much younger than you. My father is a perfect example of this. He goes to the gym regularly and plays vigorous squash a few times a week, competing successfully with good players many years his junior.

Rambam observes:

> Hippocrates said that someone who is used to a particular physical activity, even if he has a weak body or is old, is able to tolerate it better than a young strong person who is not used to this activity.[14]

Elsewhere, Rambam writes:

> As to what you mentioned, that you feel weak after exercise, the cause of this is the omission of regular exercise. If you resume exercising gradually, little by little, you will achieve as much strength and vitality as one should find after any exercise that is done properly.[15]

WHAT IS THE DEFINITION OF EXERCISE?

A balanced exercise program should include the following components:

– **Cardiovascular exercise.** This is the centerpiece of any exercise program. This type of exercise works the heart and lungs continuously, and increases oxygen consumption. Exercises that fall into this

14. *Commentary on Hippocrates' Aphorisms* 2:49.
15. *Causes of Symptoms* 18.

category include brisk walking, jogging or running (treadmill or outside), hiking, stair climbing, rowing, swimming laps, bike riding (stationary or outside), aerobic classes, skiing and jumping rope.

- **Toning and strengthening exercises.** These form an important part of any well-balanced exercise program. This type of exercise builds muscle mass and bone density, and reduces the signs and symptoms of many debilitating diseases. It also provides a significant increase in metabolic rate, which is enormously helpful for weight loss and long-term weight control.[16] Exercises included in this category are those which use weights. In addition, push-ups, abs crunches and squats are some of the most effective strengthening exercises, as they use the weight of your own body. (We will learn more about strengthening exercises in Phase 2.)

- **Stretching exercises.** These are done to warm up and cool down before and after exercising, respectively. Warming up is important for preventing injury as well as gaining maximal benefit from the exercise. An excellent way to warm up and cool down is by simply doing your cardiovascular exercise at a slower pace.

This is how Rambam defined exercise:

There are many different types of physical activities. [However,] not every body movement is considered by physicians to be "exercise."[17]

The definition of exercise is *physical movement that alters respiration*, resulting in deep breathing, and at a faster pace than usual.[18]

---

16. See second Internet reference for Phase 1, Week 2, on page 324.
17. *Regimen of Health* 1:3.
18. *Medical Aphorisms* 18:12.

> One should begin exercising slowly, increasing [the pace] until he
> reaches the optimum level of exercise.[19]

> After exercising, one should do expansion and contraction
> movements.[20]

In one of his treatises, Rambam suggests that the Sultan take a leisurely horseback ride in the morning, without stopping, gradually increasing his pace until his limbs become warmed and respiration changes.[21]

The ancient physicians stressed the importance of a well-balanced exercise program. Rambam writes that one should preferably exercise all parts of the body equally: "An exercise must move the body and its limbs moderately, each limb performing its activity so that all the parts of the body...benefit."[22]

Galen[23] wrote about an exercise which he considered to be the most effective. Regarding one of the aspects of this exercise, he says, "The vigorous part of it, which involves holding, throwing and catching, tends to tone and strengthen the body."[24]

We see from the above that the ancient physicians wrote about and promoted the three main components of an exercise program (cardio, strengthening and stretching). Yet there is still another fundamental component of exercise that is often ignored today. The following mind-boggling excerpts were written by Rambam:

19. Ibid., 18:14.
20. Literally: Make consistent movements and reverse movements; see *Medical Aphorisms* 18:15, trans. Fred Rosner (Haifa: The Maimonides Research Institute, 1989).
21. *Causes of Symptoms* 21.
22. *Medical Aphorisms* 17:4.
23. Galen lived from 129 to about 210 CE. He is considered the most important physician after Hippocrates, who laid the foundations of rational medicine.
24. *Galen: Selected Works*, pp. 299–304 (exercise with the small ball).

> The best type of exercise is that which influences the soul and causes it to rejoice.

> Happiness alone has cured or at least made milder many physical and psychological ailments.[25]

> One should pay more attention to exercise of the soul than exercise of the body. All types of exercise should always result in happiness, delight and rejoicing.[26]

Here Rambam mentions the subject of psychosomatics explicitly. This is the scientific study of the intricate interconnections between mind and body, and how it affects human health and disease.

Today, so many people get caught up in the physical effects of exercise alone. However, while the physical aspects of exercise are essential, the psychological effects should not be overlooked. Interestingly, the connection between exercise and psychological well-being has been documented. The American Heart Association states that physical activity reduces feelings of depression and anxiety, improves mood and promotes a sense of well-being.[27] The Centers for Disease Control and Prevention states:

> Physical activity and mental health epidemiologic research among men and women suggests that physical activity may be associated with reduced symptoms of depression, clinical depression, symptoms of anxiety, and improvements in positive affect and general well-being. In general, persons who are inactive are twice

25. *Medical Aphorisms* 18:2.
26. Ibid., 18:3.
27. See third Internet reference for Phase 1, Week 2, on page 324.

as likely to have symptoms of depression than are more active persons.[28]

Regular physical exercise stimulates the central nervous system, which increases the transport of oxygen to the brain as well as cerebral metabolic activity of various neurotransmitters including dopamine, serotonin, norepinephrine, and acetylcholine. Furthermore, a recent study found that participation in an exercise training program was comparable to treatment with an antidepressant medication (a selective serotonin reuptake inhibitor) for improving depressive symptoms in older adults diagnosed with major depression.

While the relationship between mind and body has only truly been acknowledged in the last twenty years by the medical world, it was already well-known to many of the great ancient doctors such as Hippocrates and Galen.[29] However, none of the ancient doctors stressed or developed the subject of psychosomatics as Rambam did. In fact, one of the most famous physicians and historians of Cairo concludes his biography of Rambam with a famous poem which describes Rambam as a healer of the "body and mind," as opposed to Galen who was mainly a physician of the body. Rambam's works are filled with explicit discussions of psychosomatics.

28. U.S. Department of Health and Human Services, *Physical Activity and Health: A Report of the Surgeon General* (Atlanta: U.S. Department of Health and Human Services, Centers for Disease Control and Prevention, National), Chapter 4, "The Effects of Physical Activity on Health and Disease, p. 136. The fourth Internet reference for Phase 1, Week 2, on page 324 cites all the relevant research.
29. Hippocrates believed that emotions were merely the consequences of the interaction between the "four humors": Black bile, yellow bile, phlegm and blood. Later, Galen recognized that emotions played a more prominent role, and so he introduced the concept of the "non-naturals" into the equation (see Chapter 1).

WHEN IS THE BEST TIME TO EXERCISE?

Rambam writes, "The general rule is that the best time to exercise is at the beginning of the day, after a person wakes up[30] and before he eats."[31] Elsewhere, he says that it is proper to eat only *after* moderate exercise.[32]

From Rambam's different writings, it seems that there are two reasons why it is best to exercise specifically before eating:

1. Exercise after eating is unhealthy

2. Exercise before eating has special advantages

Regarding exercise after a meal, Rambam writes:

> Exerting yourself after a meal ruins the digestion[33] and can lead to serious illness.[34]

> Just as movement before meals is completely good, movement after meals is completely bad...[35] because the food is being digested in the stomach and it can spread through the body prematurely without having been digested sufficiently.[36]

Exercising before meals is actually hinted to in the verses, "By the sweat of your brow will you eat bread" (*Bereishis* 3:19) and "Bread of laziness you shall not eat" (*Mishlei* 31:27).[37]

Earlier, we learned that exercise improves and strengthens our digestive systems. It seems that this benefit is enhanced if the exercise is done before

---

30. *Regimen of Health* 1:3.
31. *Mishneh Torah, Hilchos De'os* 4:2.
32. See *Medical Aphorisms* 17:11.
33. *Treatise on Hemorrhoids* 1:5.
34. See *Mishneh Torah, Hilchos De'os* 4:3.
35. See *Regimen of Health* 1:3; *Medical Aphorisms* 17:1.
36. See *Treatise on Asthma* 5:5.
37. *Kitzur Shulchan Aruch* 32:6.

meals. Yet it is very possible that you do not have to do a full workout to gain this particular benefit of exercise. As Rambam writes:

> One should not eat until one takes a walk or exerts oneself in some other way, to the point where the body *begins to warm up.*[38]

Anyone who exercises knows that this stage occurs closer to the beginning of a workout, about five minutes after starting to exercise. Rambam's use of the phrase "begins to warm up" is not just a slip of the pen, because he is always extremely careful with his word choices. There are other places when he discusses "exercising a lot."[39] Therefore, it would seem that simply raising the body's temperature is enough to gain the benefit of exercise. So taking a very short walk or doing some basic strengthening exercises before a meal could really improve the way your body metabolizes the food you eat immediately afterwards.[40]

I know someone who is fit and slim, and who often runs on the spot for a hundred counts before he eats!

What other times are good for exercising?

Rambam writes:

> Otherwise, the best time to exercise is after the complete digestion of the evening meal, so that one will be ready to receive food anew the next morning.[41]

---

38. See *Mishneh Torah, Hilchos De'os* 4:2; *Kitzur Shulchan Aruch* 32:6; *Treatise on Hemorrhoids* 1:5.
39. *Mishneh Torah, Hilchos De'os* 4.
40. This is also apparent from Berachos 23b, which Rabbi Yosef Kapach suggests is the source of this Rambam. The Talmud talks about walking ten times four *amos* or four times ten *amos* (approximately seventy feet). Either way, this is not a long distance. Rambam does not explain this source the way other commentaries do, i.e. that the purpose of this walk is to bring on the elimination process.
41. *Medical Aphorisms* 18:13. See also *Regimen of Health* 1:3 and *Treatise on Asthma* 5:5.

You should wait at least two to three hours after a meal before exercising. (Note: Exercise increases the metabolic rate, so if it is done too close to bedtime you may have a hard time falling asleep. If this is the case, exercise before dinner.)

In general, it is best to exercise at a set time each day, so that a habit is formed. It is harder to maintain a program if the exercise is done "whenever you are free," because as we all know, we seldom seem to be free!

SOME PRACTICAL SUGGESTIONS

Let us end off by offering some ideas for maintaining an exercise program:

- **Do it the same time every day**. This can be difficult, but once you get used to exercising at the same time every day, skipping a session will feel like you left something behind!

- **Do it first thing in the morning**. If you push off exercising for later on in the day, you stand the risk of missing your workout. As the day progresses, responsibilities increase and we all get weary. Exercising in the morning injects us with energy and helps us begin the day on a very positive note.

- **Keep the program simple and practical.** Do not make unrealistic, grandiose goals.

- **Switch exercises if you are not enjoying it**. Remember, if you are not happy, you will ultimately fail. The emotional effect of exercise is extremely important. If you do not enjoy doing the same exercise every day, you can alternate between various cardiovascular exercises. You could take a fast-paced walk outside on one day, participate in an aerobics class the next day and cycle on a stationary bike the following day.

- **Do something you enjoy while exercising**. For example, listen to music while you exercise to make it more pleasant for you. This adds to the psychosomatic effect of the exercise.

- **Exercise with a friend or at the gym**. If you find it hard to start or continue an exercise program, do it with a friend or join a gym. This will help you to get motivated, and you might make a good friend!

- **Choose an "at home" sport**. For those of you with a limited amount of time each day or for bad weather days, it is crucial to have an indoor exercising option. A stationary bicycle, a treadmill or a mini trampoline are good options when you can't "shlep" outside. Today, you can also buy reasonably priced basic strengthening exercise equipment for home use.

As you see, you do not need a very complicated workout, nor do you need that much time, to attain all the benefits of exercise! Is one and a half to three hours a week out of a 168-hour week asking too much for all of the amazing benefits that come from exercising?

Exercise is not a luxury! It is fundamental to our health.

Let me stress the most important thing: Get up and DO SOME EXERCISE, even if it is just for a few minutes! Most times, the hardest part is putting on those walking shoes or getting onto that bicycle or treadmill. Put some enthusiasm into it; once you start, you're on your way! In fact, when you get going, you will feel so good that you will often have to stop yourself from overdoing it! In the beginning, it's not so much about the workout itself but about habituating yourself to an exercise program. While not always noticeable at first, it is the small steps which build the solid foundation that you need.

In Phase 2, I will discuss cardiovascular and strengthening exercises in more detail. At that point, I will show you exactly how to go about building the exercise habit in a practical way.

PHASE 1 / WEEK 2
PRACTICAL METHOD

YOUR SECOND WEEK

In addition to your High-Water-Content Meal once a day, you will begin with five to ten minutes of cardiovascular exercise, five times a week.

While this may seem like a drop in the bucket, it is very significant because you are laying a solid foundation for a well-balanced exercise program in the future.

At first, stick to cardiovascular exercises. These include: brisk walking, jogging or running (on a treadmill or outside), hiking, stair climbing, rowing, swimming laps, bike riding (stationary or outside), skiing and jumping rope. Basic strengthening exercises will be introduced in Phase 2.

Obviously, you do not have to build up slowly if you are already following a well-balanced exercise program. Continue with your existing schedule or switch to the final stage of our basic exercise program, which consists of fifteen to twenty minutes of cardiovascular exercise and some strengthening exercises including push-ups, sit-ups and squats, five times a week.

For those of you who are not exercising at the moment, this is the best way to start: Do five to ten minutes, five times a week, and enjoy it! Remember to exercise before meals and try to set a fixed time for your exercise program. By the end of Phase 2, you will be following a well-balanced exercise program.

Gabi from South Africa lost 18 pounds – exercise secrets

I have always been more serious about my exercise than my diet. That is why people often ask me for advice about a practical exercise program. In the past, I used to suggest various exercises but generally, the people I tried to help could not sustain the complicated, time-consuming workouts. Now I suggest the basic, well-rounded exercise program of the Life-Transforming Diet, and I can see the relief on their faces. I have noticed that they stick to the program because they are able to slowly build up, adding exercises when they are ready for them.

I have also been motivated to follow the Life-Transforming Diet's eating program. The combination is MAGIC! I have realized that the key is not complexity but simplicity and practicality.

Yosef from Israel – Classical writings

It was interesting to read how many profound principles of Rambam are intertwined with the writings of classical Mussar teachers in this book. This whole program is a system for successful control of eating habits, but it has relevance for the successful control of any aspect of our lives – emotional, physical and psychological. Rambam's teachings about health really come to life in this book. I have seen a change in my eating habits and I also have a much better understanding of my emotional development and habits.

PHASE 1 / WEEK 3

Method "Substitution" between meals

Continue – High-Water-Content Meal once a day

– Five to ten minutes of cardiovascular exercise five times a week

THE SNACKING CHALLENGE

Perhaps the worst contravention of the Food Quantity principle is the snacking that most people do between meals. Snacks add up, and little bites or nibbles throughout the day also add up! That means that we may actually be eating four or five meals a day – or more! Furthermore, snacks are often of poor nutritional value.

The cycle of snacking perpetuates itself because it ruins your natural appetite for the main meals. This may well be the reason why so many children eat poorly at mealtimes.

Interestingly, when Rambam discusses how a teacher should motivate children to study, he writes:

> The teacher should tell the student that he will give him nuts, figs or a little honey.[1] One cannot expect a child to study for the sake of knowledge itself.

Besides the insightful educational message here, it is interesting to note what people considered to be a treat in those days. Imagine the average,

---

1. Note the stress on "a little" honey, and the fact that it is at the end of the list. Rambam taught (*Mishneh Torah, Hilchos De'os* 4:12) that honey is in general bad for children.

present-day kid getting motivated by a nut, a fig or a little honey! In sharp contrast, today we are bombarded with enticing, convenient, cheap snacks and junk food.

Rambam begins his famous chapter on health[2] with the following principle:

> A person should eat only when he is hungry and he should drink only when he is thirsty.

Notice how in one line Rambam sums up the crux of the issue. We have to learn *when* to eat and when to drink. If we do this, we will be left feeling truly satisfied and our unhealthy cravings will automatically diminish.

Nonetheless, the snacking challenge is certainly not an easy one! Most popular diets do not really deal with this issue, and it can be particularly difficult when we are already at our correct weight. While losing weight we have a clearly defined goal, but maintaining our success is a constant battle. Without the necessary tools and knowledge, it seems that we are bound to fail.

I am certainly not going to suggest that all snacking between meals is out of bounds. I am saying that we must learn when to snack and on what to snack. In this way, we can save our bodies from immeasurable harm, and we will actually be improving our health, weight and energy levels.

What is the secret of achieving this?

To control a craving we need to zone into its true source. We need to know how to tell the difference between a craving and genuine hunger.

---

2. *Mishneh Torah, Hilchos De'os* 4:1.

CRAVINGS VERSUS NATURAL HUNGER

Read the following brilliant insight:

> A genuine desire for food occurs when one is hungry because the stomach is empty, but a craving is a longing for a specific food.[3]

After being stated so clearly, this seems so obvious!

Animals in their natural habitat never overeat or indulge in addictive behavior. In fact, a deer will walk calmly in front of a pack of lions that have already made their kill. The deer instinctively knows that a lion will not eat more than it needs.[4] However, if a piece of chocolate could walk, it probably would never venture close to a person, even if that person had already eaten a scrumptious, filling meal!

Is it possible that animals have more control than you or I? Or could animals perhaps be "wired" differently than human beings? Read about the following experiment.

A group of three-year-olds were given very large portions of macaroni, yet ate only as much as they were hungry for. But a group of five-year-olds ate more when given larger portions. Does this mean that three-year-olds have more control than older children and adults?

According to Barbara Rolls, Ph.D., of Pennsylvania State University, learned behavior overtakes instinct between the ages of three and five. While the body instinctively would stop eating when satisfied, we *learn* to choose the biggest piece of cake or to "clean our plates."[5] Thus, overeating has nothing to do with control. *A craving does not satisfy any real need.* In fact,

---

3. *Kitzur Shulchan Aruch* 32:10.
4. See also *Michtav Me'Eliyahu*, vol. 1, p. 39.
5. Dr. Howard M. Shapiro, *Picture Perfect Weight Loss: A 30-day Plan* (Emmaus, PA: Rodale Books, 2002), p. 23.

sometimes we experience a craving even after eating a satisfying meal. This cannot just be about enjoyment! Do we really enjoy stuffing down more food on top of more food? If we are honest with ourselves, we will admit that we do not actually need the food we crave. Our apparent need is only an illusion.[6]

Another proof is that our cravings never seem to be alleviated. "Just one more chocolate," we tell ourselves, "Just one more piece of cake." Yet we aren't satisfied by giving in. Cravings do not satisfy any real lack, so they continue unabated.

Regardless of whether the source of a craving is emotional or superficial, the common denominator is that the object we crave has no real intrinsic value to us. It will not remove the cause of or deal with the problem. So even when we have eaten what we craved – and more – it almost always leads to a feeling of frustration, sadness or sometimes even depression.

In contrast, true hunger is the result of a physiological need to fill your stomach. It is an amazing stimulus, intended to remind you to fulfill your nutritional requirements.[7] *Hunger is a real need.* Its source is in an actual internal deficiency. You can push it off only for a limited amount of time. Eventually you will either have to eat something or you will simply die.[8]

Therefore, when you get hungry, it is not that you crave a specific food. Rather, you want food in general, in order to satisfy hunger's natural calling.

---

6. See *Michtav Me'Eliyahu*, vol. 1, author's note, p. 42.
7. Ibid., author's note, p. 41.
8. King Solomon seems to substantiate this fundamental principle: "The righteous person eats to satisfy his soul, and the belly of the wicked will want" (*Mishlei* 13:25). In light of our discussion, this statement comes to life. We are being told: A person who eats in order to satisfy the source of his physical well-being will be satisfied. He has responded to a real physiological need. However, someone who eats simply because that is what his belly craves at that moment, will never be satisfied (see Malbim on the above verse). Similarly, Rambam writes, "A person who is ruled by his appetites will never be satisfied from following his desires" (see *Mishneh Torah, Hilchos De'os* 1:1).

Having satisfied that need, you will no longer want to eat. After all, the goal has been accomplished! This also explains why an animal or a three-year-old instinctively stops eating when satiated. Their natural hunger has been satisfied.

What we have discussed about food cravings holds true about other cravings as well – both physical and emotional. Cravings manifest themselves in almost every aspect of our lives, and we usually fool ourselves into thinking that attaining the desired object will bring us the illusive happiness we so desire. We rarely even enjoy the coveted prize we achieve. Instead, we invariably get trapped in a net of never-ending cravings.

With food, the problem is often magnified because the natural hunger urge can get entangled with our cravings. This makes it very difficult to differentiate between true hunger and cravings. As a result, we do not know when to stop – not only when we snack, but even when we are hungry and eating in order to fulfill a perfectly natural physiological need.

It is important to stress the following point: While the source of a craving is sometimes very strong, it is only through *habit* that any craving truly gains momentum. The intricate mechanism of habit formation intensifies and entrenches cravings. Eventually, a "need" is born to constantly satisfy our unhealthy cravings. Clearly, reshaping our habits is crucial when it comes to our relationship with food.

SWEET TOOTH

If unhealthy cravings are simply an illusion, why do most of us crave specifically sweet foods? Why do we avoid foods which are sour or bitter?

We were given an amazing, built-in warning system, better known as taste buds, which protect us from "bad" foods and slant us toward "good" foods.

Rambam writes regarding quality of food:

> In general, one should not eat foods whose bitterness or sharpness is apparent, or those foods that are very sour.[9]

> One should always try to eat dishes that are sweet or that have only just a little sourness.[10]

> Cooked food that has been left until it smells, or any food that has a bad odor or is very bitter, is like poison to the body.[11]

Taste buds warn us that moldy, sour or bitter foods are bad for us. They also send a message that sweet foods are good for us. Becoming aware of this helps us appreciate the miraculous workings of our body and teaches us to listen attentively to its signals.

In truth, our taste buds are more than just a warning system. Rambam writes that people were created in such a way that positive actions result in pleasure. This serves as an incentive to do them.[12] We were given an incentive to do the things which we need to do anyway. Thus, certain foods taste delicious and make us feel good as an incentive for us to eat the right types of beneficial foods. In fact, Rambam writes that one of the criteria for good-quality food is that it be enjoyable to eat.[13]

What sweet foods are among the healthiest foods? The answer is fruit and sweet vegetables. They taste delicious and invigorate our bodies. Many health studies have shown that fruits and vegetables can help prevent various serious illnesses. In fact, the National Cancer Institute states:

---

9. See *Treatment of Hemorrhoids* 1:2–3.
10. *Causes of Symptoms* 20.
11. *Mishneh Torah, Hilchos De'os* 4:9.
12. Commentary on *Mishnah Sanhedrin* 7:4.
13. See *Regimen of Health* 1:2.

People whose diets are rich in fruits and vegetables have a lower risk of getting cancers of the colon, mouth, pharynx, esophagus, stomach, and lung, and possibly prostate cancer. They are also less likely to get diabetes, heart disease, and hypertension. A diet high in fruits and vegetables helps to reduce calorie intake and may help to control weight.[14]

The Talmud says that it is forbidden for a scholar to live in a city that does not have its own source of vegetables[15] or certain fruits.[16]

Thus, there are two sides to a craving. There is the illusory or unhealthy craving for sweet-tasting non-nutritious foods, and there is the genuine or healthy craving for sweet nutritious foods. Perhaps this is why cravings are so enticing, because we really do physically crave sweet things.

Unfortunately, the pleasure and taste of food, which was designed to be an incentive or warning system for us, has now become a gateway to obesity and illness. Through technology and processing techniques, many unhealthy, cheap and bitter foods have been transformed into sweet-tasting foods. *We have created an artificial experience that imitates the intended beneficial experience of enjoying tasty food.* Therefore, our goal must be *to reinstate the integrity of our natural internal systems.*

I believe that the most effective solution for controlling our bad cravings is to actively feed our good cravings. In this way we will automatically be substituting our artificial cravings for what our sweet tooth really wants and needs. That is why I call this method *Substitution*. Through it, we are preventing our cravings from gaining a foothold.[17]

---

14. For more information, see the Internet reference for Phase 1, Week 3, in Appendix E (page 325).

15. *Eruvin* 55b. Rashi says because they are healthy and inexpensive.

16. *Sanhedrin* 17b.

17. *Chovos HaLevavos, Sha'ar Yichud HaMa'aseh,* Chapter 5, explains that this is the only way to uproot the inclination to overindulge.

SUBSTITUTION

In the Substitution Method between meals, the first preference is drink, the second preference is vegetables, the third preference is fruit and the fourth preference is nonfat milk products within certain guidelines. Let's take a look:

Drink

First of all – and this is very important – what you may think is hunger between meals may really be thirst. So before you eat anything between meals, first drink something, preferably water.

Water is the most beneficial beverage for the body.[18] Inexpensive, natural and refreshing, it is far healthier than any other drink, even if that drink is calcium- or vitamin-enriched. In fact, every cell in the body needs water to function. Without water, we would die in a few days.

Rambam writes:[19]

> The physicians have already listed some of the [amazing] benefits that result from drinking a moderate amount of water:
>
> – Water strengthens all the internal organs.
>
> – Water improves digestion and adjusts the stomach for food.
>
> – Water improves one's physical appearance.
>
> – Water helps prevent certain illnesses.
>
> – Even a small amount of water quenches thirst.

18. See *Kitzur Shulchan Aruch* 32:17.
19. *Treatise on Asthma* 7:3–4.

▮ — Clean water helps maintain our correct body temperature and it also speeds up the elimination cycle.[20]

Regarding water quality, Rambam writes, "The best quality water is clear, light, tasteless and odorless."[21]

From a weight-loss perspective, water has been shown to assist in losing and maintaining weight loss. Some people make the mistake of thinking that drinking less water will help prevent water retention. The opposite is true. Drinking more water stimulates the kidneys, which actually helps reduce water retention.

It is important to drink at the right time. When is the best time?

The best time to drink is between meals. It is good for your health and excellent for controlling your cravings. As Rambam writes,[22] "[The best

---

20. See *Kitzur Shulchan Aruch* 32:17.

21. *Medical Aphorisms* 20:38. See also *Treatise on Asthma* 7:3 and *Regimen of Health* 4:14. This is what Rambam has to say about water quality:

> Rainwater [is best because it] does not putrefy quickly. If you cannot find rainwater, spring water is satisfactory if it is pure and clean. (*Medical Aphorisms* 20:36)
> The poorest quality water comes from melted snow or ice because it never returns to good [quality] rainwater. (*Medical Aphorisms* 20:33)
> When bad waters that are turbid or putrid are boiled and then filtered of dust particles, they become appropriate for drinking. (*Medical Aphorisms* 20:37; see also *Treatise on Asthma* 7:3)

This is what Rambam has to say regarding water temperature:

> Lukewarm water weakens the body, ruins one's constitution…. One should be extremely careful to avoid this type of water. (*Treatise on Asthma* 7:4)
> Cold water, which is not as cold as ice, is the best type of water and it should be drunk when one is thirsty. (*Treatise on Asthma* 7:3)
> Water which is not cool is extremely harmful to the digestion of all people…and even a large quantity fails to quench one's thirst. (*Treatise on Asthma* 7:3)
> Water should not be too cold, as it delays digestion and the elimination cycle. (*Medical Aphorisms* 20:34)

22. *Mishneh Torah, Hilchos De'os* 4:2. Rambam says that one may drink a small quantity of wine during the meal (ibid.). One may also drink a small amount of cold water during the

time to drink is] when the food begins to be digested." Elsewhere, he defines this time as about two hours after the meal.[23] At the very least, one should wait at least one hour after the meal.[24] Rambam held that drinking right before a meal or drinking a large amount during the meal is harmful.[25]

There is no need to set specific amounts to drink. Rambam tells us that a person should drink only when he is thirsty.[26] It is not good to drink too much water. As Rambam writes, "For some people, drinking a lot of water is harmful."[27] However, the fact is that many people ignore their natural urge to drink, or they respond either by eating or by drinking the wrong beverages. Therefore, the following guidelines will insure that you are drinking enough water during the day.

- You should try drinking two cups of cool or hot (not lukewarm) water in the morning after you wake up.

- Between breakfast and lunch, you should try drinking another two cups of cool or hot water.

- Between lunch and dinner, you should try drinking another two cups of cool or hot water.

This regimen alone can transform your life. You will feel better and more energetic throughout the day, your health will improve and you will gain much better control of your cravings.

You certainly do not need to drink more than the above amount of water per day. This is because we are eating enough high-water-content foods

meal (see *Regimen of Health* 1:4), if drinking with your meals agrees with your constitution (see *Treatise on Asthma* 7:3).
23. *Treatise on Asthma* 7:3.
24. See *Treatise on Hemorrhoids* 1:4.
25. *Medical Aphorisms* 20:32; *Mishneh Torah, Hilchos De'os* 4:1–2.
26. *Mishneh Torah, Hilchos De'os* 4:1.
27. *Regimen of Health* 4:8.

every day, at our HWC meal and sometimes between meals. These foods also supply the body with pure water.

While water is always the best choice, I will list other drinking options in this week's "Practical Method" section below. But whatever else you drink, it should preferably supplement but not replace your regular water consumption. No drink can compare with or replace the amazing benefits of plain water.

SOME THOUGHTS TO PONDER ABOUT SODA

The Center for Science in the Public Interest (CSPI) reports that government data shows that the average twelve- to nineteen-year-old American male drinks more than two cans of soda per day, about *868 cans of soda annually*. The average American female in that same age group consumes 1¾ cans a day. Overall, Americans are consuming twice as much soda as they did twenty-five years ago, spending about $54 billion a year on it. That's twice what Americans spend on books.

Here are just a few facts about soda:

- Each 12-ounce can of soda contains between seven and twelve teaspoons of sugar. Artificial sweeteners such as aspartame, saccharin and acesulfame potassium are added to diet sodas.

- The caffeine added to so many drinks is one of the best ways to insure you that you will return for more.

- Sodium benzoate-E211 and potassium benzoate-E212 are used both as food preservatives and to disguise taste in poor-quality food. They may cause nettle rash, aggravate asthma and give allergic reactions. Besides these, there are other additives put in your favorite sodas. Check the label.

Continued on next page

> – Most sodas include many different types of acid, like malic acid E-296 which can be either synthetic or derived from fruit. These give your dentist a lot of business.

Food

What happens if you quench your thirst between meals but still feel hungry? Whenever you want to eat something between meals, begin by eating some non-starchy vegetables. Try strips of cucumber and red pepper with some added herbs. Steamed vegetables are another popular option. You can find a list of all the non-starchy vegetables at the end of Chapter 13.

You may also eat *medium*-starchy vegetables such as beets, butternut squash, carrots, pumpkin and peas. I call these medium-starchy vegetables because they are higher in carbohydrates and calories than non-starchy vegetables. However, I group them with vegetables because they have about half the carbohydrates and calories of regular starches such as potatoes and rice. So you could also eat sweet baby carrots, add butternut squash to a vegetable soup or eat the latter alone between meals.

If you are in the mood for something sweeter instead, eat a piece of fresh fruit. Many health professionals maintain that a person can benefit most from the healthy properties of fruit if it is eaten on an empty stomach.[28] Indeed, as we mentioned in Phase 1, Week 1, Rambam already understood this principle over eight hundred years ago: "One should eat fruit only on an empty stomach",[29] "One should never combine fruit with a meal.[30] Thus, eating fruit as a snack between meals is a perfect time. (Rambam writes

28. See Phase 1, Week 1.
29. See *Treatise on Asthma* 3:9.
30. See *Regimen of Health* 1:13. See also *Causes of Symptoms* 10–11 and *Mishneh Torah, Hilchos De'os* 4:6.

that a small quantity of constipating fruits such as apples may be eaten immediately after the meal.[31])

Rambam and many health professionals maintain that in general, one should wait at least two to three hours after a meal before eating again.[32]

How much fruit can you eat between meals? As long as it is within reason, I don't think it's necessary to limit fruit quantity. This is especially true in the beginning Phases, when most people's between-meal eating habits are poor. Remember, if you drink first, you will not need to eat that much in order to satisfy a craving between meals. In general, one fruit between meals should eventually be enough. Vegetable assortments are even better between meals. High in fiber and low in calories, they are virtually impossible to overeat.

On occasion, your sweet tooth may not be satisfied with a fresh fruit. Try a little natural dried fruit (no added sugar). Quantities should be watched carefully because dried fruit is highly concentrated. For example, you may have two or three medium dates, one or two dried figs, a one-ounce (28g) package of raisins, two or three prunes or four or five pieces of dried mango. This is usually more than enough to satisfy a sweet craving. These quantities constitute about a one-ounce serving of dried fruit.

What happens if you drink water and are still hungry, but are simply not in the mood for vegetables or fruit?

It is important to realize that although a food may be "healthy" or "nutritious," any food between meals – except fruit and vegetables – is still considered an exception because it can end up being an extra meal. However, there *is* a nutritious and low-calorie option which is easily

---

31. *Causes of Symptoms* 11; *Mishneh Torah, Hilchos De'os* 4:6.
32. See *Regimen of Health* 1:4; *Treatise on Asthma* 6:3,7:3; *Mishneh Torah, Hilchos De'os* 4:1,5; *Kitzur Shulchan Aruch* 32:6.

digested and will neither ruin the balance of your two main meals a day nor increase unhealthy cravings.

I am talking about nonfat milk products. The key is *nonfat*, because regular milk products are high in saturated fat and calories. In Chapter 13, we will see that saturated fat cannot be used positively by the body at all.

Rambam writes:

Galen writes that milk is more nourishing than wheat.[33]

The best and thinnest milk is goat's milk, and cow's milk is also good.[34]

The best type of fresh cheese is that which is made from milk whose fat has been removed. This cheese is one of the most satisfying of all types of cheeses, digests quickly and provides good nourishment.[35]

In contrast, Rambam writes regarding full-fat cheese:

It is well-known that cheese is a fattening, thickening food, and when it is old it is extremely bad.[36]

Cheese is among the foods that should be eaten only periodically and in small quantities.[37]

Therefore, you may add the following foods as a "fourth preference" in the Substitution Method.

---

33. See *Medical Aphorisms* 20:40.
34. However, see *Medical Aphorisms* 20:43 in the name of Galen, but see also *Medical Aphorisms* 25:10 and 25:30.
35. See *Medical Aphorisms* 20:45.
36. *Treatise on Asthma* 3:4.
37. *Mishneh Torah, Hilchos De'os* 4:9–10.

1. Nonfat and certain low-fat yogurts

   – Serving size: 6 oz. (170 g) container. Usually between 60 and 100
     calories (251–418 kilojoules) per container. (The nutrition label located
     on most packaged food products will be discussed in Chapter 13.
     Depending on the country in which you live, you will find nutrition
     data listed in calories, kilojoules, or both. One calorie = 4.184 kilojoules,
     so 100 calories is about 418 kilojoules.) If there are more calories, you
     can be sure that there is a large amount of added refined sugar or that
     the portion is too large.

   – Fruit yogurt is not a good option, as fruit should only be eaten on an
     empty stomach. Plain yogurt is preferable, but you can get vanilla and
     other flavored yogurts which fall within the guidelines above.

2. Nonfat or low-fat cottage cheese

   – Serving size: ½ cup (114 g) – 80 to 90 calories.

   – In this case, low-fat cottage cheese is also an option because it has
     about the same calories per serving as nonfat cottage cheese and only
     10 calories are from fat.

3. Nonfat string or sliced cheese

   – Serving size: the equivalent of 80 to 90 calories

   – Nonfat is especially important when it comes to cheese. The fat
     content of low-fat cheese is still high. For example, a serving size
     (1 ounce or 28 grams) of low-fat string cheese has 80 calories, 45 of
     which come from fat.

4. Nonfat or very low-fat milk

   – Serving size: 1 cup (8 fl. oz.) – 90 calories.

   – If you are unable to get zero percent milk and therefore must drink 1
     or 2 percent, try to limit it to a 6-fluid-ounce serving instead.

You will notice that I mention "calories." This does not mean that you should become obsessed with calorie counting. The point is that we do not want these snacks between meals to ruin the balance of your two main meals a day. (In Phase 1, Week 5, you will see that eating larger amounts of dairy products with vegetables would be considered a Light One CF Meal.) The nonfat milk products option, when limited to 90 calories, insures that we will not overstep the healthy snack boundaries between meals, and it is not even considered an exception. Most nutritionists agree that 90 calories of food is a very acceptable snack between meals. In fact, many fruits have an equal calorie count. For example, one medium size apple (5½ oz.) has 90 calories.

The only other time that I ask you to pay attention to calories in this system is when you are comparing non-nutritious foods. It follows that you are better off indulging in a lower calorie non-nutritious food than a high calorie non-nutritious food. Otherwise, nutritional content always takes precedence over calories. This subject will be discussed in detail in Chapter 13.

So why can't I eat any food that is less than 90 calories between meals? you might be thinking. With most other foods, it is very hard to limit quantities. Also, many snacks which people think are healthy are in reality high in sugar, saturated fats or trans-fats. Some examples are most crackers, cookies, potato chips and chocolate. At this stage, the risks are too high. The above options offer natural, very nutritious, and high-calcium foods. However, once you are at goal weight, you will have the option to make "Smart Exceptions," which allow for almost any food between meals.

The nonfat/low-fat milk products option also has an important psychological element. It insures that we do not overeat the wrong foods between meals just because we are in the mood to eat something else besides fruits and vegetables.

IMPORTANT: If you eat one of the nonfat dairy options between meals, you should not eat fruit. Fruit must be eaten alone. You can still eat vegetables, because they mix with all foods except fruit.

Try to prepare your between-meal plan. You don't want to be stuck without the means to satisfy a craving in a nutritious way. Stock up on vegetables and fruit, as well as nonfat dairy products.

As time passes, cravings for the wrong types and amounts of food will decrease. Gradually new, good habits will replace the old, bad ones. In fact, many people find that they no longer even enjoy the oversweet, artificial taste of their old cravings after getting used to the real thing!

AVOIDANCE

How is it that some people succeed in transforming their homes so that even the children change their eating habits? A lot of it has to do with their making a technical change, for at the beginning, no deep behavior modification takes place.

We all know that one of the most effective ways to deal with unhealthy cravings or non-nutritious foods is to avoid them. This is not only logical; it is simply the way the mind works. Why? In general, even the strongest cravings start off being weak. As long as the source of the craving is somewhat removed, the instinctive process of "craving" will not be significantly aroused. Consequently, the most effective and easiest way to deal with unhealthy cravings or non-nutritious foods is by removing yourself from all contact with them.[38] The old adage sums it up beautifully:

---

38. See *Cheshbon HaNefesh*, Chapter 13, "*Perishus.*"

"Out of sight, out of mind." What your eyes do not see, you eventually will not crave.

This is especially true for those who spend a large part of the day in the house. At home, the nibbling can go on endlessly. Therefore, avoid bringing home the products that you do not want to eat. Just as an alcoholic or a smoker must remove all the products that feed his addiction, so too, should we remove the unhealthy foods that we crave.

Avoidance really begins at the supermarket. Before shopping for groceries, make a list – and stick to it! And never go shopping when you are hungry, so that you can think with your head and not with your stomach and eyes!

Clean out your food cupboards and pantry. It's time to rid yourself of all the foods you no longer want around you. Some households naturally resist this measure. I can fully understand that! Try to explain to your family members that it is all about habit. You are not trying to convince them to completely give up their favorite treats. In fact, there is still room for "Smart Exceptions" once you are at goal weight. However, haphazard exceptions can only lead to health and weight complications. It is always best to eat treats out of the house.

Once you are ready for "Smart Exceptions," if you are going to allow them at home, it is important to buy single serving pack sizes. It is much harder to limit yourself to one or two scoops of ice cream from a tub than it is to eat an ice pop or small cup of ices. Likewise, when you finish one small package of baked potato chips, it is finished. Try stopping when you are in the middle of a large package of chips and you'll see what I mean! With single serving size snacks, you know that when you are finished, *it is over*! And you can relax, knowing that you really enjoyed your allowed snack.

It is best to make healthy changes in the household while the children are still very young. Show your love for them by making the choice to improve the quality of their lives. Childhood obesity is becoming a bigger and bigger problem (excuse the pun). The best solution is to prevent the problem from the start.

The older members of the family will probably come to understand the benefits of a healthy diet themselves. Still, people resist change...at first. So be patient. Hopefully over time, they will all begin to appreciate your point of view – not only for your sake, but for theirs as well.

There are some households that are particularly resistant to change. If you find yourself in such a situation, perhaps everyone can agree to keep unhealthy foods inaccessible to you so that a spur-of-the-moment craving will probably have dissipated by the time you can get your hands on the item you crave.

It definitely helps to have a large supply of delicious looking fruit and vegetables in the house. Encourage good habits with the right foods! Most important, be a good role model. When your family observes you eating healthily and correctly and they see how wonderful you look and feel, they will want the same for themselves!

A particularly vulnerable and challenging time is the weekends, namely Shabbos. Remember that cakes and candy do not fit into the guidelines of the Substitution Method. Concentrate on your meals, and be prepared to implement Substitution between meals. Smart Exceptions will be introduced when you are at goal weight.

PHASE 1 / WEEK 3
PRACTICAL METHOD

YOUR THIRD WEEK

In addition to your High-Water-Content Meal once a day and
five to ten minutes of cardiovascular exercise five times a week,
you will begin the Substitution Method between meals.

If you are eating your main meals properly and snacking on the right foods
between meals, you should always feel satisfied and never hungry at any
point. The keyword here is "hungry."

At first, it is only natural to experience some cravings between meals,
but it is important not to confuse this with hunger. These are *habitual*
cravings, which have been established over time. Please do not fall into the
common trap of thinking that giving in to an unhealthy craving will satisfy
it. On the contrary, giving in actually *feeds* the power of a craving.[39] As
Rambam writes, one intends to satisfy his thirst but thereby intensifies it.[40]

The good news is that as strong as a craving may be, it is short-lived. No
matter how urgent it may seem, it's only a momentary illusion. So if we can
hold out for just a few minutes or divert our attention away from it, the
strength of the craving will diminish and eventually disappear completely.
When you feel a craving, immediately implement the Substitution Method.

---

39. See Ramban (*Devarim* 29:18, s.v. *lema'an sefos*), who writes that this principle also
applies to eating habits.
40. *Shemoneh Perakim*, end of Chapter 3.

The Substitution Method

This is the order of preference between meals:

First preference

- Always try to begin with water. If you want to add a bit of "zing" to the taste, add a slice of lemon. Have hot water if you prefer it. You should drink two cups of water in the morning after you wake up, another two cups between breakfast and lunch and two more cups between lunch and dinner.

- While some naturopaths are not in favor of seltzer (soda water), it is definitely the closest "fizz drink" to water. You may also have water or seltzer with added natural flavor (zero calories).

- Herbal tea is another option.

- Caffeine-free coffee or diet soda (see footnote, below[41]).

Second preference

- If you are still not satisfied after quenching your thirst, eat some fresh or steamed strips of vegetables with added herbs. You may eat non-starchy or medium-starchy vegetables. You may also make vegetable juice.

---

41. The health-conscious may be shocked by this suggestion. Interestingly, the "health" of these products is a bitter debate among the professionals. It is probably best not to drink these beverages and certainly not to start the habit. That is why they are at the bottom of the list. But we cannot deal with everything simultaneously. We are not keen to give too many No's at once. If you are used to drinking diet soda or coffee, I do not think that this is necessarily the best time to stop. It is often much easier to cut back or eliminate these products after the Phases (see end of Chapter 11). Everyone agrees that being overweight or obese is extremely dangerous, and we are focusing on reducing that danger.

Or Third Preference

– If you are in the mood for something sweeter, eat some fresh fruit instead of the vegetables.

– If this does not do the trick, eat a little natural dried fruit, preferably about a one-ounce serving.

Or Fourth Preference – nonfat/low-fat dairy products

– Check that it has approximately 90 calories (or less):

  • 6-oz. container of nonfat or low-fat yogurt (you may have up to 100 calories of low-fat yogurt)

  • ½ cup nonfat or low-fat cottage cheese

  • nonfat string or sliced cheese

  • 8-oz. cup of nonfat milk or 6-oz. glass of very low-fat milk

– These are options only if you have not used the fruit preference.

At this stage, do not drink any commercial fruit juices. In general, limit the amount of any fruit juice. It lacks the fiber advantage of whole fruits, and you may inadvertently be *drinking* large quantities of fruit. Remember – no refined sugar drinks. If you drink coffee or tea, add one or two teaspoons of sugar or honey only. If you want milk in your coffee or tea, try to use nonfat milk, although 1 percent is also acceptable.

Keeping the house full of nutritious foods and empty of non-nutritious foods can literally transform your household. Breaking the habit of buying non-nutritious food can be hard, but it is certainly much easier than saying No in the midst of a craving when your cupboards are stocked with "the bad stuff."

It is important to try to stick as closely as possible to the clear guidelines listed above. Read the four preferences the Substitution Method offers over again. Be careful not to "cut and paste" your own choices. There are many options within the guidelines, and their clarity will give you peace of mind.

If you still feel "hungry" after going through all the stages of Substitution, you can be absolutely sure it is not hunger that you are experiencing. Let me put it bluntly: *It is time to close your mouth and take a breather.* Get on with other things you want to do or have to do. Give yourself the opportunity to break the shackles of your unhealthy cravings and habits! At this stage of the program, you will have basically removed any other foods from the realm of your food choices between meals.

INSIGHTS AND SUCCESS STORIES

Malki from England lost over 30 pounds – an end to unhealthy snacking

I used to snack a lot between meals without even being aware of it. I snacked on things such as chocolate, pastries, fruit leather, rolls, chips and nuts. If it was there, I'd eat it. Now I've become more conscious of what I put into my mouth. Resisting temptation was difficult at first, but has now become second nature. The Life-Transforming Diet works with a system of behavior modification, and it has helped me "transform" my relationship with food.

PHASE 1 / WEEK 4

Method   Main One-Concentrated-Food (One CF) Meal

Continue – High-Water-Content Meal once a day
             – Five to ten minutes of cardiovascular exercise five times
               a week
             – Substitution Method between meals

THE OVEREATING EPIDEMIC

Obesity is the result of a complex interaction of social, behavioral, cultural, environmental, physiological and genetic factors.[42] The focus of this chapter is the relationship between overeating and obesity.

Short-term overeating is a common human habit. However, when it is sustained over long periods, it becomes a real health risk. Long-term overeating will always lead to body fat storage and obesity. In other words, *overeating ultimately makes you obese and keeps you obese!*

> Obesity meets all the accepted definitions of "disease" on the basis of generally accepted scientific evidence…. [It is] recognized as a disease by agencies and officials of the United States government [and] world health organizations…as well as by [over nine] major non-governmental medical and scientific authorities.[43]

42. In Appendix E (page 325), you will find a list of all relevant Internet sources backing up the facts and statistics stated in this section.
43. See third Internet reference for Phase 1, Week 4, on page 325.

Most of us feel totally helpless and hopeless when it comes to the quantity of food we consume at a meal. It seems that once we are seated at a table, we become victims of the contents of that meal. Moreover, overeating often becomes addictive.[1]

Truthfully, we are not entirely to blame – bigger quantities have become the norm. In Western societies, active overeating is generally driven by marketing factors. Food sales are promoted on the basis of quantity-for-money rather than quality-for-money. These values often become ingrained in the culture. For instance, visitors to the United States are invariably shocked by what they see as excessive portion sizes served at food outlets. However, these same portions are accepted as the norm by native citizens.

For example, "super size" is a hefty portion, but even the regular size is big enough to satisfy more than one person! In fact, in the last twenty years, the standard size of a hamburger has increased 112 percent. Bagels are 95 percent bigger, and servings of pasta have gone up 480 percent. Is it just a coincidence, then, that in roughly the same time period, according to United States government figures, there has been a 40 percent increase in people who are overweight and a 112 percent increase in those who are obese?

We have to learn how to let go of this overeating addiction and accustom ourselves to eat the correct quantities of food.

1.   "Overeating: The Health Risks" (see second Internet reference for Phase 1, Week 4, on page 325), quoting A. Stunkard, R. Berkowitz, T. Wadden, C. Tanrikut, E. Reiss, L. Young, "Binge Eating Disorder and the Night-Eating Syndrome," *International Journal of Obesity-Related Metabolic Disorders* 20:1–6 (1996).

OVEREATING IN THE RAMBAM

Rambam writes:

- Overeating is like poison to the body.[2]

- Even the best foods, eaten in excess, corrupt one's digestion and this can lead to illness.[3]

- The preservation of health lies in abstaining from satiation.[4]

- Overeating can lead to illness.[5]

- Satiation causes the filling of the stomach and its distention...the stomach cannot digest the food adequately at all, causing weakness, sluggish movement and heaviness from food.[6]

- When the meal is digested poorly in the stomach, inevitably the subsequent stages of digestion are also bad...because of the potentially severe harm it can cause, all physicians warned against satiation.[7]

In his *Treatise on Asthma*, Rambam mentions a very long list of physical and psychological ailments that can result from bad digestion and overeating.[8] In *Mishneh Torah*[9] and *Moreh Nevuchim*,[10] Rambam stresses the negative moral implications of overeating.

---

2. *Mishneh Torah, Hilchos De'os* 4:15.
3. See *Treatise on Asthma* 5:3. See also *Regimen of Health* 1:1.
4. *Regimen of Health* 1:1; *Treatise on Asthma* 5:5.
5. See *Commentary to Hippocrates' Aphorisms* 2:17.
6. *Regimen of Health* 1:1.
7. Ibid.
8. *Treatise on Asthma* 5:3–5:6.
9. *Hilchos De'os* 5:1.
10. 3:8, 3:35, 3:38.

OVEREATING IN CURRENT SOURCES

Rambam's view of overeating and its ramifications are substantiated by current studies and statistics.

Several years ago, the head of The American Obesity Association (AOA) urged the Dietary Guidelines Advisory Committee to "make a paradigm shift from focusing strictly on content of dietary intake to a balance of content and total quantity of dietary intake."[11] More recently, the Mayo Clinic wrote: "Just as important as what you eat is the manner in which you eat. Poor digestion may simply be due to bad habits. Moderate portions are digested more comfortably. Large meals put increased demands on digestion, since your body is only able to produce a certain volume of digestive juices."

In one study,[12] "researchers followed nearly three hundred obese and overweight adults as they entered a weight loss program. All of the participants received instruction in five different weight loss strategies: increasing planned exercise (walking), increasing regular physical activity (incidental walking associated with chores or work), cutting back on fat in the diet, eating more fruits and vegetables, and controlling portion size. After two years of follow-up, researchers found that those participants who spent the most time actively controlling portion size during their weight loss and maintenance efforts were more likely to lose weight. Practicing the other strategies also increased the likelihood of losing weight, but controlling portion size had the greatest impact. Consequently, this study shows that controlling portion size may be the single most effective thing you can do to promote lasting weight loss."

11. Press release, "Obesity Group Weighs in on Dietary Guidelines, Asks Advisory Committee to Consider Total Quantity of Foods," Washington, March 8, 1999.
12. E. Logue, "Longitudinal Relationship between Elapsed Time in the Action Stages of Change and Weight Loss," *Obesity Research*, vol. 12 (September 2004): pp. 1499–1508. News release, Summa Health System.

The American Diabetes Association states:

> More and more children are overweight or obese. Being overweight
> increases your child's risk for type 2 diabetes. The good news is
> that losing a small amount of weight can lower risk. If your child
> has diabetes and is overweight, losing weight can help lower blood
> glucose levels. If your child is trying to lose weight, it doesn't mean
> your child has to cut out favorite foods. But it is a good idea to
> reduce serving sizes. Your child can include favorite foods in a
> healthy meal and still lose weight.[13]

OVEREATING DEFINED

In *Mishneh Torah*,[14] Rambam writes, "One should not eat until his stomach
is full. Rather, [he should stop when] he is close to three-quarters satiated."
He defines overeating more clearly in three of his medical works:

> It is important to rely on the principle that a person should not
> satiate his appetite, but should rather stop eating while a little of
> his appetite remains.[15]

> Physicians have fixed appropriate limits in this matter by saying that
> a person should stop eating before he detests it, preferably when
> most of his appetite has been satisfied and only a little appetite
> remains.[16]

13. See sixth Internet reference for Phase 1, Week 4, on page 325. If your child has diabetes,
work with his health care team to develop a meal plan that is right for him.
14. *Hilchos De'os* 4:2.
15. *Treatise on Hemorrhoids* 1:2.
16. *Treatise on Asthma* 5:2.

> Satiation is eating until the appetite is removed.... Because of the
> potential harm, all physicians warn against satiation and order a
> person to stop eating while his appetite still remains.[17]

We see that Rambam makes mention of two stages in overeating –
satiation and revulsion. He writes that the correct time to stop eating is
even *before* being satiated. Thus, to preserve health and energy, we must
learn to stop eating when most of our appetite is satisfied and only a little
appetite remains.

ARE YOU OVEREATING?

Rambam puts it beautifully:

> There are some people who have a large stomach and a strong
> digestive system and they can tolerate a large amount of food.
> Other people have a small stomach and a weak digestive system
> and they can tolerate only a small amount food.[18]

Rambam also gives the following advice:

> It is well-known that the art of medicine is devised only for rational
> beings. Therefore, every person should calculate the amount of
> food which can be easily tolerated and easily digested. This should
> be done when one is healthy and it should be calculated in the
> springtime. This amount should be considered one's basic portion.

17. *Regimen of Health* 1:1.
18. *Treatise on Asthma* 5:1. See also *Commentary on Hippocrates' Aphorisms* 1:17.

One should reduce it gradually as the heat increases, and increase it gradually as the cold increases.[19]

In other words, we cannot generalize when it comes to what constitutes overeating, because everyone is different. The quantity of food I can eat will differ from how much you can eat. Still, the general principle is the same for everyone:

The main principle in this matter is to avoid harmful satiation and distention of the stomach.[20]

FINDING THE SOLUTION: THE ONE-CONCENTRATED-FOOD MEAL

So what can we do to combat our overeating challenge without resorting to weight loss pills, weighing our portions or constantly counting calories? On a practical level, how do we prevent ourselves from overeating without taking radical steps?

Rambam makes a practical suggestion, which will insure that you do not overeat and that your appetite will subside before satiation occurs.[21] He

19. Ibid. Rambam writes:
> During the winter, natural body heat is increased and the need for food is greater. (See *Commentary on Hippocrates' Aphorisms* 1:15)
> During the summer, one should eat less because the digestive system is weaker in relation to the dispersal of natural [body] heat. (See *Regimen of Health* 1:2)
> One should eat two-thirds in the summer of what one eats in the winter. (*Mishneh Torah, Hilchos De'os* 4:12)
> In the summer, one should eat cooling foods, without many spices, and use vinegar. In the winter, one should eat warming foods, use many spices, and eat a little mustard and *chiltit* [an herb]. This applies to both cold and hot climates. (*Mishneh Torah, Hilchos De'os* 4:8)

20. *Treatise on Asthma* 5:1. See also *Regimen of Health* 1:1.
21. See *Regimen of Health* 1:1.

teaches it in the name of the ancient physicians. It has many physiological advantages. This is what he wrote over eight hundred years ago:[22]

> There is a recommendation given by the ancient physicians in order to prevent overeating. One should not eat many foods at a meal. Instead, *a single (main) dish should be eaten per meal.* [The ancient physicians] give a few reasons for this:
>
> – A single food is best for digestion because there is only one stomach, and different foods digest in various ways according to the food's particular nature.[23]
>
> – When you eat a single food, you need not be concerned with the sequence of foods consumed. In some opinions, heavy foods should be eaten before lighter foods. Others disagree and hold that first lighter foods should be consumed and then heavier foods. Some opinions hold that laxative foods should be eaten before constipating foods. However, if you eat one dish, you do not have to be concerned with the above sequence.[24]
>
> – What is much more important than the above advantages is that many foods at a meal cause a person to overeat. That happens because the appetite is stimulated with every food. But with a single food, the appetite is satisfied, so that most likely you will not overeat. In any case, generally, you eat less when you eat one food than when you eat many foods. A rule for health maintenance is to eat an amount that does not allow you to reach a stage of satiation.

---

22. *Treatise on Asthma* 5:4. See also *Regimen of Health* 1:1.
23. Rambam writes, "A wise person eats only one or two foods at a meal, consuming enough to sustain himself. This is what King Solomon said (*Mishlei* 13:25), 'The righteous person eats to satisfy his soul.'" (See *Mishneh Torah, Hilchos De'os* 5:1.)
24. See also *Mishneh Torah, Hilchos De'os* 4:7.

In his *Treatise on Asthma*, Rambam writes regarding this principle:[25]

> Many physical and emotional symptoms develop from bad digestion. Some include heartburn, insomnia, melancholic distress, pain in the colon, intestines, joints etc.... Intelligent healthy people should contemplate whether the pleasure they derive from eating justifies all those ailments...which can be avoided if one limits the meal to a single good food, does not fill oneself with it and does not exercise after eating it.... If this precaution is indispensable for healthy people, how much more should it be obligatory for ill people.[26]

To sum it up, these are the advantages of eating a single dish according to the Rambam:

1. The food is digested well, according to its particular nature.

2. We do not have to pay attention to the sequence of foods consumed.

3. Many physical and psychological ailments that may develop from bad digestion can be prevented.

4. The appetite is not overstimulated. This prevents overeating at the meal.

5. It's easier to prepare (my wife said I should throw this one in!).

I like to call this method the One-Concentrated-Food (One CF) Meal. We already mentioned that "concentrated foods" include all foods besides fruits and vegetables. Fruits and vegetables are considered "high-water-content foods."[27]

---

25. See *Treatise on Asthma* 5:3–5:6.
26. See *Treatise on Asthma* 5:3–5:7.
27. Concentrated foods such as starch and protein take much longer to digest, requiring from two to six hours and sometimes more. Compare this to high-water-content foods such as fruit and vegetables, which take from twenty to sixty minutes to digest.

When Rambam lists the "main foods," he mentions only concentrated foods such as proteins and grains.[28] Thus, it appears that he is referring to a concentrated food for the "one" main food at a meal.

Therefore, the One CF principle says that a meal should consist of either a protein or a starch for the main dish. At a One CF meal, you cannot eat from both of these food groups. However, you can always eat non-starchy or medium-starchy vegetables with your concentrated food, and it is still considered a One CF meal because these vegetables mix well with all concentrated foods. So as a side dish, choose sautéed, steamed, grilled or raw non- or medium-starchy vegetables. [Use minimal amounts of oil when sautéing. Non-stick sprays are preferable. Heating fats will be discussed in Chapter 13.] Butternut squash, acorn squash, spaghetti squash, pumpkin and peas are medium-starchy vegetable options. They are a great substitute for regular starch side dishes such as potatoes and rice. (See a full list of foods and food groups at the end of Chapter 13.) Remember: Fruit should not be eaten at a meal.

In Phase 3, "Mixed Meals" will allow any number of foods, even from different food groups, at the same meal. Shabbos meals and the like will be discussed below.

TAKING SECONDS

Although certain food combinations are not allowed, the One CF Meal is a wonderful option because you do not have to be as careful with quantities and it does not lead to feelings of deprivation. Rambam does not give actual quantity limits with this method. On the other hand, its main advantage is that one will not overeat. Isn't this a contradiction?

28. *Regimen of Health* 1:6.

Rambam is teaching that the One CF method results in the natural shrinking of your appetite. In other words, when you digest food properly and your appetite is not overstimulated, you will *naturally* stop before satiation occurs. In time, you will no longer overeat at the meal.

Therefore, you may want to take extra helpings of the concentrated food at this meal. This is normal in the beginning especially, because many people are used to overeating or eating the wrong foods at a meal. Moreover, one cannot generalize when it comes to portion size. No one is the same, and everyone has different requirements. This does not mean that you *must* take seconds, but if that is what you want, do not hold back. Allow your body to return to its natural integrity.

With the One CF principle, the main dish can be really enjoyed and savored. Furthermore, even if you do overeat at a One-Concentrated-Food meal, the excess food can be digested more efficiently and you will certainly feel the difference. Just use some common sense so that you do not leave the meal feeling heavy or sick.

THE SCIENCE OF FOOD COMBINING

Today, food combining is a hot topic of debate. There are many health professionals who swear by it. Dr. William Howard Hay introduced food combining to United States in 1911, and Dr. Herbert M. Shelton made it famous. Many bestselling books have been written and many health organizations have been set up based on their principles.

In a nutshell, this is the main principle: Protein digests in a more acid environment and carbohydrates in an alkaline environment. If you combine them at a meal, the hydrochloric acid neutralizes the more alkaline ptyalin. As a result, the starches start to ferment and the protein putrifies. This can cause allergies, gas, heartburn, and headaches, among other symptoms. Furthermore, the food takes much longer to digest. This requires a lot more energy.

In contrast, correct food combining results in increased energy levels, better assimilation of nutrients, better digestion and a decreased appetite. This leads to weight loss and better weight maintenance.

However, there are also many health professionals who disagree with the whole concept of food combining. Their argument is that combining protein with carbohydrates slows down the sugar release from foods into the bloodstream. Thus, combining them has the advantage of stabilizing blood sugar levels and consequently, weight control. Yet interestingly, even many of these professionals agree that food combining is probably best for those with digestive problems.[29]

This type of disagreement is certainly not unusual in the field of nutrition. One thing is clear, however: According to Rambam, eating only one concentrated food at a meal is best for digestion. And as I mentioned above, most people seem to agree on this point. Still, the most important aspect of this method, says Rambam, is that it prevents both the overstimulation of the appetite and overeating. This can also be verified through experience. And since overeating is probably the greatest factor leading to obesity, clearly the One CF method can be very effective in insuring the maintenance of weight.

Nevertheless, in Phase 3, you will have the choice to eat a "Mixed Meal." Rambam was not necessarily opposed to mixing protein with starches at a meal. He just believed that the One CF principle was the *optimum* way to eat. Still, from Phase 3, you can enjoy the advantages of combining protein and starches at a meal. In other words, from Phase 3, you can choose to be somewhere in the middle of the two modern-day opinions mentioned

29. Patrick Holford, *The 30-Day Fat Burner Diet*, 4th ed. (London: Piatkus, 1999), p. 18.

above. One main meal a day can consist of both protein and starches (Mixed Meal), and one main meal a day would consist of either protein or starches (One CF Meal).

CONCENTRATED FOODS WITHIN THE SAME FOOD GROUP

Is it still considered a One CF Meal if you have more than one concentrated food within the same food group? For example, if you eat two protein foods such as fish and chicken or feta cheese and fish at the same meal, would this still be a One CF meal?

Strictly speaking, this would not be considered a One CF meal. After all, you are eating more than one concentrated food. However, you would not necessarily lose all the advantages of the One CF method. In other words, it is probably better for the digestive system than eating both protein and starches at the same meal, because you are eating foods within the same food group.

Interestingly, naturopaths believe that it is best not to mix proteins, because each type is of such different composition that they digest differently. However, this only applies to two different categories of proteins such as flesh proteins, eggs, nuts and dairy products. Thus, two different types of *flesh* proteins or two different types of nuts may be eaten together. Regarding starches, everyone agrees different types may be eaten together because they are much easier to digest. So you could eat bread with potato or beans with rice.[30]

30. *Fit for Life*, p. 54.

Nevertheless, according to Rambam, there are two caveats to bear in mind if you choose to eat a second concentrated food within the same food group. First and most important, you should limit the quantity of the second concentrated food, because if you eat a big quantity of both foods you will most likely risk overstimulating the appetite, which defeats the main purpose of this method. Secondly, the sequence of concentrated foods consumed may become an issue, as Rambam writes:

> When a person wants to eat chicken and meat at the same meal, he should eat the chicken first. Similarly, [if one wants] eggs and poultry (at the same meal), he should eat the eggs first. Small cattle should be eaten before large cattle. A person should always begin with the lighter food and then proceed to the heavier food.[31]

DESSERT OPTIONS

Rambam writes:

> A small amount of constipating fruits such as pomegranates, quinces, apples and [crustumenian pears] can be eaten after the meal in an amount that will strengthen and close the mouth of the stomach.[32]

A small amount of unsweetened applesauce is a popular dessert option. Homemade always tastes better. Constipating fruits include apples, bananas, pears, pomegranates and quinces. Rambam says that fruit eaten at the end of a meal should be eaten in small quantities. So eat cut-up pieces,

---

31. *Mishneh Torah, Hilchos De'os* 4:7. Notice that Rambam mentions only concentrated foods regarding the correct order of consumption.
32. See *Regimen of Health* 1:13. See also *Causes of Symptoms* 10–11 and *Mishneh Torah, Hilchos De'os* 4:6. See also *Treatise on Asthma* 3:9–10.

preferably half a fruit but not more than a whole fruit. The equivalent in applesauce is from a quarter to half a cup. Remember, if you are hungry before eating the fruit, you could take seconds of the main concentrated food or the high-water-content side dishes.

At this stage, we are sticking to fruit for dessert because we are removing our unhealthy cravings. Completely natural, these foods do not feed bad cravings. Other options are introduced when you can better differentiate between a healthy and unhealthy craving. In Phase 3 there are many low-calorie refreshing dessert options such as dairy, ice, gelatin and Tofutti frozen products. Nuts and certain candies will also be options. After you are down to your desired weight, you will even have the option to eat any dessert within certain guidelines, as will be discussed in Chapter 11.

EATING OUT

The beauty of the Life-Transforming Diet is that you do not have to retreat from your life in order to succeed. For example, the Main One CF Meal is extremely easy and practical when you eat out. At a restaurant, order your favorite steak, grilled chicken, grilled fish or any other main protein dish. Have grilled vegetables or a salad to go with it. Plain vegetable soup (without added creamer or MSG) is an option. It is always a great starter.

Even fast-food outlets have a variety of Main One CF meals. Chicken or fish is usually the safest. The quality of the red meat options may not be the best at those venues. Remember, fried food is like poison to the body, and salad drenched in regular dressing can be very fattening. Order plain salads as a side order and add your own low-fat or nonfat dressing. (Food quality will be discussed in detail in Chapter 13.)

If you enjoy wine, drink a glass of unsweetened wine with your main course. Rambam writes, "One may drink a small quantity of wine during the meal."[33] Moreover, in the Talmud,[34] it says that wine is the greatest of all medicines and in a place where there is no wine, drugs will be necessary. Rambam writes that wine is beneficial for the body and the soul. He mentions many benefits of drinking wine (in moderation and at the correct time) throughout his medical and other writings. For instance, "If wine is consumed properly, it is a major factor in the preservation of health and the cure of many illnesses."[35] On our program, you may drink one small glass (about 4 oz.) of unsweetened wine per day, but preferably not more than five times a week.[36]

MAIN ONE CF MEAL ON SHABBOS

The Friday night Shabbos meal will be your main meal on Friday. Shabbos day lunch will be your main meal on Saturday. While it is hard to make these meals a strict Main One CF Meal, you can still try to keep to some of its guidelines. As I mentioned before, Shabbos is a day on which there is a special mitzvah to enjoy food. On the other hand, the authorities write that it is not a time to cultivate bad eating habits or to overeat.

During the Friday night meal, it is best to try sticking to the main protein dishes and vegetable side dishes. As Rambam writes, the less variety of foods you eat, the less your appetite will be stimulated. This is also

33. *Mishneh Torah, Hilchos De'os* 4:2. One may also drink a small amount of cold water during the meal (*Regimen of Health* 1:4), if drinking with your meals agrees with your constitution (*Treatise on Asthma* 7:3).
34. *Bava Basra* 58b.
35. *Regimen of Health* 4:10. See also ibid., 1:10; *Treatise on Asthma* 7:1; *Commentary to Hippocrates' Aphorisms* 2:18; *The Art of Cure* (Rambam), chapter 7.
36. People with medical issues should obviously consult their doctor concerning the consumption of wine.

preferable from a digestive point of view because it will leave you (and your stomach) feeling better after the meal.

It is important to pace yourself through the courses. Eat one piece of fish and if you want, have some plain vegetable or chicken soup. In between, eat salad or vegetable side dishes and chew properly.[37] Most important, focus on the company of your family and friends! Speak to them instead of eating more. Notice that by the time most people reach the main course they are so full that they are not really able to even enjoy it! By following the Life-Transforming Diet guidelines, you will be able to savor the main course of chicken or meat and fulfill the mitzvah of *oneg Shabbos*. (Notice how the order of foods consumed in a traditional Shabbos meal is also in line with Rambam. As we learned, he writes that if one eats more than one concentrated food at the same meal, he should start with lighter foods.[38] Therefore, fish should be eaten before chicken or meat, which is the usual order of a Shabbos meal.)

It is preferable not to eat any condiments such as mayonnaise, nor to eat kugels and starchy side dishes. If you really feel you must do so, *on an occasion*, then keep it to an absolute minimum and choose nonfat or low-fat products. Remember to make vegetable side dishes an important part of the meal. If the meal is continuing for an extended period of time and you feel like reaching for more food, take salad or vegetables. They will keep you satisfied until the next course.

Bear in mind that some salad dressings are extremely fattening and unhealthy, so be on your guard. Certainly when you are at home, change to fat-free or low-fat dressings, or make your own with olive oil, lemon juice

---

37. Ben Ish Chai (*Parashas Emor*) suggests that you put down the cutlery or food between bites. This way you can concentrate on the food in your mouth instead of the food on your fork or in your hands.
38. *Mishneh Torah, Hilchos De'os* 4:7.

and spices. Salads do not have to drown in dressing – it is only there to enhance the taste!

It is obligatory to eat bread at the first two Shabbos meals. But you should not eat more than one thin slice of challah (the size of a slice of white bread), which is more than a *kebeitzah*. This fulfills all aspects of the obligation.[39] Chew your challah slowly and enjoy it! It is a very good idea to take the challah off the table after everyone gets their piece, or at least remove any other pieces from in front of you.

You may drink a small glass of dry red wine during the meal. Limit the drinking of any soda or even water to a minimum during the meal, as Rambam writes that it can hinder digestion.

Dessert options have been discussed in detail for each Phase. Some people skip dessert altogether. But if you choose to eat some dessert, in Phases 1 and 2, you can choose a small amount of constipating fruits such as apples or plain applesauce, or pears (see page 149 for a list of these fruits). In Phase 3, you may choose low-calorie desserts. After you are at goal weight, you may eat any dessert as a High-Cal Exception.

For the Shabbos day meal, simply follow the same guidelines as the night meal. The Life-Transforming Diet guidelines apply to all special occasions or celebrations where there is usually an abundance of food with numerous courses. Just stick to the protein and vegetable side dishes and pace yourself carefully. If you frequently find yourself at these kinds of occasions, it can certainly take its toll on even the firmest of resolves to eat healthily. So follow our guidelines and partake of the function's delicious and permitted foods without guilt and regrets!

If you are going to eat starches at the Shabbos day meal such as the barley and potatoes in the cholent, then pay special attention to the Mixed Meal

---

39. See Appendix D.

guidelines (introduced in Phase 3), or do not eat the proteins such as fish, chicken and cholent meat at this meal. A pareve cholent is a delicious alternative to a meat-and-grain one. It is especially important not to burden your plate with piles of food. At a Mixed Meal, you may only take seconds of salad and vegetables. If you are going to have fish, eat one piece. Remember to eat only one slice of bread and follow the other guidelines mentioned above. Keep the words of the *Shulchan Aruch* in front of you: "A wise man plans ahead by not filling his stomach."[40] Gross overeating (*achilah gasah*) is not considered eating.[41]

Keeping to our guidelines insure that you will fulfill the mitzvah of enjoying the Shabbos meals, walk away without feelings of guilt or lethargy and still continue on your journey to weight maintenance and optimum health.

40. *Shulchan Aruch, Orach Chaim* 291:1.
41. *Mishnah Berurah* 291:4.

PHASE 1 / WEEK 4
PRACTICAL METHOD

YOUR FOURTH WEEK

In addition to a High-Water-Content Meal once a day,
five to ten minutes of cardiovascular exercise five times a week,
and the Substitution Method between meals,
you will begin eating a Main One-Concentrated-Food (One CF) Meal.

The One CF principle says that a meal should consist of either a protein or a starch for the main dish. You should not eat from both food groups at the same meal. However, you can eat any vegetable side dish (high-water-content food) with your concentrated food and it is still considered a One CF Meal. (Fruit should not be eaten at a meal.)

Most people prefer to eat chicken, fish, meat or a soy product as a main dish at their biggest meal of the day. In the Life-Transforming Diet, this meal would be a Main One CF Meal. In the United States, most people eat this meal for dinner. In Europe and Israel, many people eat this meal for lunch. The remaining main meal is usually a lighter meal. In our system, this would be a Light One CF Meal, introduced in Week 5, which consists of lighter proteins such as eggs, feta cheese, flesh protein toppings such as sliced grilled chicken or tuna on a salad, OR starchy carbohydrates such as bread, pasta, rice and potatoes.

There is almost nothing like a good barbeque, but you can roast, boil or steam your food. No deep frying. As a side dish, choose sautéed, steamed, grilled or raw vegetables. Medium-starchy vegetables such as butternut squash, acorn squash, pumpkin and peas are also an excellent side dish option. Plain vegetable soup is always a good starter.

Most people prefer a flesh protein as the concentrated food at this meal. It is generally more filling, and it often prevents snacking on the wrong foods between meals. I definitely think it is worth spending the extra money on these foods, because your health and weight maintenance are priceless! Nevertheless, if you eat light protein at the Light One CF meal, you may choose to make your Main One CF Meal a starch meal. You could eat bread, grains such as rice, millet, quinoa or barley, pasta with a tomato-based sauce, potatoes or sweet potatoes – with a salad or vegetable side dish. If you desire, you may eat different starches at the same meal. Whole wheat options are preferable.

Butter (whipped, "light" butter), avocado or olive oil (cold-pressed) may be used sparingly as a spread or topping. Other examples of starch meals will be presented in the next chapter. For most people, it is a good idea to limit bread and grains to one meal a day.

Most modern health professionals suggest that we eat fish at least twice a week and limit eating red meat to twice a week. Similarly, Rambam writes, "One should try not to eat even of the best types of meat unless one becomes bored with chicken."[42] For the sake of variety, it is a good idea to plan your meals throughout the week to use different proteins and/or starches.

Remember, you can take extra portions at this meal. But although you don't need to stint on the portions, you certainly don't want to leave the meal feeling sick. In time, your appetite will return to its natural integrity.

---

42. *Causes of Symptoms*, point 20. See also *Mishneh Torah, Hilchos De'os* 5:10.

At this stage, dessert options include unsweetened applesauce or a small amount of constipating fruits. Other dessert options will be introduced from Phase 3.

Remember not to eat dinner too close to bedtime. Rambam writes that one should wait three to four hours after a meal before going to sleep.[43]

INSIGHTS AND SUCCESS STORIES

Dana from United States – over the moon

I haven't been able to wear fashionable clothing for years, but now I can choose from a variety of styles. When I went clothes shopping this time, I had to ask the saleswoman for a smaller size! My husband is also thrilled with my progress. I'm still in the early stages of the Life-Transforming Diet, and I'm already seeing marvelous results. Thank you for writing this book!

Nechama from the United States lost 17 pounds – Shabbos meals

The best part for me is that I don't dread Shabbos meals. I follow the Life-Transforming Diet plan: I think it through beforehand. I eat my slice of challah – SLOWLY – and enjoy it. I have a small piece of fish, the salads, vegetables and the main course. No kugel – and if I choose to, I have more salad. I enjoy my food. I don't feel deprived. I focus more on the company than on the food.

The same applies to eating out. I order whatever protein I want – grilled – and a salad. I check that the salad dressing is low-fat, and I don't even miss the chips or the oily vegetables. I don't order dessert because I am so happy with the way I look that I refuse to jeopardize my success so far.

43. *Mishneh Torah, Hilchos De'os* 4:5.

PHASE 1 / WEEK 5

Method   Light One-Concentrated-Food (One CF) Meal

Continue   – High-Water-Content Meal once a day
– Five to ten minutes of cardiovascular exercise five times a week

– Substitution Method between meals
– Main One-Concentrated-Food (One CF) Meal for the main meal

LIGHT ONE CF MEAL

The Light One CF Meal is simply a lighter version of the One CF Principle. How does it fit into Rambam's diet?

We saw from Rambam's writings[44] that most people eat two main meals a day, but a healthy strong person can fulfill his main nutritional needs with one main meal a day and a second lighter meal. So while Rambam is certainly not against eating two main meals a day, he seems to be saying that the optimum for a healthy person is to eat one regular main meal and a second lighter main meal. In the Life-Transforming Diet, a Main One CF Meal or a Mixed Meal is considered the heavier main meal, and a Light One CF Meal is the second lighter main meal. In Phase 3, you will have the choice to drop one of the One CF Meals from your meal schedule.

At the Light One CF meal, you could eat lighter proteins such as eggs, or a protein topping such as fish, chicken or white cheese on top of a salad. Or

---

44. *Treatise on Asthma* 6:1.

this meal can be a good opportunity to eat starches such as bread, pasta, rice or potatoes.

Let us take a better look at the three main variations of the Light One CF Meal.

1. The Tasty Tub Version

In this option, protein is eaten as a topping on a large salad. I call it a Tasty Tub meal, and it is a firm favorite on the Life-Transforming Diet.

Use a large variety of vegetables in your salad such as lettuce, tomatoes, red peppers, carrots and sprouts. You can also add butternut squash, broccoli, cauliflower, beets and green beans.

Canned fish (packed in water) is a good protein topping. Another quick option is feta cheese or a generous helping of low-fat cottage cheese. (If you want, you could add sunflower seeds to a dairy salad.) If you are at a restaurant, most main dish salads such as a Greek salad or salad nicoise are good choices. (If the salad usually comes with a starch such as croutons or potatoes, simply ask the waiter or waitress not to add them to your salad.) Grilled chicken breast cut into thin slices is my personal favorite. Strips of baked or grilled fish is another delicious possibility.

A convenient way to take lunch to work or eat on the go is to put it into a plastic tub. That is why this Light One CF choice is called a Tasty Tub! Actually, I enjoy eating from a large, tub-like dish even when I am at home because it insures that I will make this meal a large and filling one! Give yourself a generous salad and topping – don't deprive yourself with very small portions.

Add a fat-free, low-fat or homemade dressing to the Tasty Tub. Chew slowly so you can enjoy the different flavors, and you will be satisfied when it is finished. This mix will provide you with the nutrients, vitamins, antioxidants and fiber needed in your diet. It also supplies enough protein to satisfy you until the next meal but you will still feel light and energetic for the rest of the day. Those who have tried it agree that it helps control unhealthy cravings both at the meal and between meals. This is especially important in the beginning stages of this program, when natural inner controls have not yet been re-instated.

The only difference between the Tasty Tub meal and the Main One CF Meal is that there is a higher ratio of vegetables to protein. You do not want to eat two large main flesh protein meals a day.

2. The Light Protein Version

Eat a vegetable omelet or scrambled, boiled or poached eggs with a tossed salad or strips of vegetables. (If you want, you could add some nonfat cheese to your omelet.) A salad with a cheese topping also falls into this category, but since it is mainly salad, I listed it with the Tasty Tub version.

3. The Grain Version

Rambam considered whole wheat bread to be a nutritious food. There is a mistaken impression that all bread makes you fat. In truth, many bread options are extremely healthy and non-fattening. The best kinds of bread are light whole wheat bread, a wrap, crisp bread and pita. (See Chapter 13 for Rambam's thoughts on bread, and for more bread choices and guidelines.)

Here are some examples of a Light One CF Grain Meal:

For breakfast, you could have bread toasted with some cut-up strips of vegetables or served with a regular salad.[1] You can use butter (whipped, "light" butter) or avocado as a spread on the bread, but use sparingly.

A delicious, satisfying and low-calorie lunch option is a grilled vegetable wrap or an assorted salad in a pita with some added fat-free dressing. A slice of vegetable pizza without cheese is another choice available in many fast food restaurants.

Another option is hot cereal cooked with water, or pasta with a tomato-based sauce. There are many good tasting whole wheat pasta brands.

Potatoes eaten with some olive oil or butter is also considered a Light One CF Grain Meal.

Remember, if you are not satisfied with one starch, you could eat two starches at the same meal. For example, you could eat a large salad with fat-free dressing together with crisp bread and a baked potato. Some people like a sweet potato with rice and a salad. Corn on the cob with bread is another option. There are many different starch choices and combinations (see the end of Chapter 13 for a full list of foods and food groups).

Although it is always good to eat vegetables with a concentrated meal, the Light Protein and Grain versions of the Light One CF Meal do not need to be eaten with vegetables. The Tasty Tub version aims for a higher ratio of vegetables because regular flesh proteins can be eaten in this version.

Hot cereal cooked or eaten with milk, a meat or egg sandwich, pasta with a cheese topping and a baked potato with sour cream are all considered

---

1.   The Talmud (*Bava Metzia* 107b) states that it is good to eat "a mouthful" of bread in the morning – see page 89 and the corresponding footnote. (Clearly, the bread the Talmud is referring to is nutritious, whole wheat bread without added oil or sugar.) Interestingly, Rambam does not mention this *gemara* in his writings..

"Mixed Meals" because they contain both a protein and a starch. Mixed Meals will be introduced in Phase 3.

Almost every one of these options is a popular choice at most restaurants.

What about taking seconds at the Light One CF Meal? It is best to have more salad or vegetables before taking seconds of the protein or grains. However, if you want more of the one concentrated food, go for it. Don't feel deprived and don't stint. The One CF method does not restrict quantities. Eventually, you will automatically stop eating when you are satiated.

LIGHT ONE CF MEAL ON SHABBOS

In Week 4, I said that the Shabbos Friday night and Saturday lunch meals will loosely follow the guidelines of either a Main One CF Meal or a Mixed Meal. You may eat an HWC Meal at either *melaveh malkah* or *seudah shelishis*.

The remaining Saturday meal will be your Light One CF Meal. If you did not overeat at lunch, it is probably best to make *seudah shelishis* the Light One CF Meal from a halachic point of view. This is because this meal is one of the obligated three meals on Shabbos.

As I mentioned, regarding *seudah shelishis* and *melaveh malkah*, there is a difference of opinion whether someone overweight, or concerned about their weight, must eat bread at these meals (see Appendix D and ask your Rav). But if you *do* eat bread, one thin slice fulfills your obligation according to all opinions. If you are eating bread, then make this Light One CF Meal a grain version. You could have a grilled vegetable wrap or an assorted salad in a pita with some added fat-free dressing. You could also eat other starches at this meal such as sweet potatoes or other grains.

If you would rather have protein at this meal, then you could certainly have a Tasty Tub or Light Protein version of the Light One CF Meal. Just be especially careful to limit the challah to one thin slice, as explained above.

It is important to remember why we want to be healthier and look our best. It is more important to us than indulging in our old bad eating habits. Relinquishing the tyrannical hold of overeating is especially hard over the weekend. Try to focus on your ability to choose not to be a victim of this challenging time.

PHASE 1 / WEEK 5
PRACTICAL METHOD

YOUR FIFTH WEEK

In addition to a High-Water-Content Meal once a day,
five to ten minutes of cardiovascular exercise five times a week,
Substitution Method between meals,
and the Main One CF Meal,
you will begin eating a Light One-Concentrated-Food (One CF) Meal for
the remaining meal.

As we already mentioned, the One CF principle says that a meal should
consist of either a protein or a starch for the main dish. You should not eat
from both food groups at the same meal. Vegetables (non-starchy and
medium-starchy) can be eaten with all concentrated foods.

In practice, there are three main variations of the Light One CF Meal:

1. The Tasty Tub version

2. The Light Protein version

3. The Grain version

At this point you will be eating *one* High-Water-Content meal, *one* Main
One CF Meal and *one* Light One CF meal.

INSIGHTS AND SUCCESS STORIES

Sam from the United States – Phase 1

The Life-Transforming Diet is a breath of fresh air. It did not begin with impersonal and demanding rules and regulations. It really speaks to me as a person. In Phase 1, I only had to make one lifestyle change per week. I was scared in the beginning that there were not enough stringencies for me to lose weight. Yet I could feel that things were changing: my eating habits and my relationship to food were different. And these positive changes happened at a non-threatening pace.

Ari from Israel – gradual implementation

I like the gradual implementation of the Phases. It's not overwhelming. It's exciting to start something new each week, especially because the whole program is done gradually. I like my fruit meal, and I really look forward to exercising for ten minutes without feeling guilty that it's not enough. The Light One CF Meal is a favorite of mine. I'm really only at the beginning stage, but I'm confident about transforming my life this way.

Liron from South Africa – revolutionize

I believe this book will revolutionize the way people relate to food and ultimately to themselves. Through following this program I am starting to see how my eating choices impact me on a physical, moral and spiritual level.

SUMMARY / PHASE 1

THE PHASE

Week 1

High-Water-Content Meal once a day

Week 2

Add: Five to ten minutes of cardiovascular exercise five times a week

Week 3

Add: Substitution Method between meals

Week 4

Add: Main One CF Meal at the main meal

Week 5

Add: Light One CF Meal at the remaining meal

DAILY REGIMEN

Meals

- High-Water-Content Meal
- Main One CF Meal
- Light One CF Meal

Between Meals

- Substitution Method – four preferences

Exercise

- Five to ten minutes of cardiovascular exercise five times a week

A SAMPLE DAY IN PRACTICE

The Life-Transforming Diet is not about specific foods. It is about re-educating ourselves about *how* to eat all our regular foods.

At the end of each Phase, I will show you what your day could look like depending on when you set your particular meal and exercise schedule. Our aim is to empower you to make your own choices! I have also included examples of between-meal options, based on our principles.

Below you will find three examples of what your day might look like at the end of Phase 1.

If you made breakfast your High-Water-Content meal and you did your exercise between lunch and dinner:

Upon Awakening

Two glasses of water

Breakfast – HWC MEAL

Bowl of mixed fruit with a topping of nuts

Mid-Morning Snack – SUBSTITUTION METHOD

Two glasses of water

Wait at least ten minutes, and then eat vegetables with half a cup of low-fat or nonfat cottage cheese

Lunch – LIGHT ONE CF MEAL

Tasty Tub version: Salad with protein topping

Exercise – EXERCISE PROGRAM

Wait at least two hours after lunch and do five to ten minutes of cardiovascular exercise

Two glasses of water

Mid-Afternoon Snack – SUBSTITUTION METHOD

Hot drink and fruit

Dinner – MAIN ONE CF MEAL

Grilled flesh protein dish with steamed vegetables and an optional small glass of unsweetened wine

If you made lunch your High-Water-Content meal and you did your exercise between lunch and dinner:

Upon Awakening

Two glasses of water

Breakfast – LIGHT ONE CF MEAL

Light Protein version: Vegetable omelet made with a slice of nonfat cheese and a salad

Mid-Morning Snack – SUBSTITUTION METHOD

Two glasses of water

Hot drink and fruit

Lunch – HWC MEAL

Vegetable soup and large mixed vegetable salad with nonfat dressing

Exercise – EXERCISE PROGRAM

Wait at least two hours after lunch and do five to ten minutes of cardiovascular exercise

Two glasses of water

Mid-Afternoon Snack – SUBSTITUTION METHOD

Nonfat yogurt and sweet baby carrots

Dinner – MAIN ONE CF MEAL

Grilled flesh protein dish with steamed vegetables and an optional small glass of unsweetened wine

Dessert: Unsweetened applesauce

If you made dinner your High-Water-Content meal and you did your exercise before breakfast:

Upon Awakening

Two glasses of water

Exercise – EXERCISE PROGRAM

Five to ten minutes of cardiovascular exercise

Breakfast – LIGHT ONE CF MEAL

Grain version: Toast with strips of vegetables (millet, quinoa or another grain may also be eaten)

Mid-Morning Snack – SUBSTITUTION METHOD

Two glasses of water

Hot drink and fruit

Lunch – MAIN ONE CF MEAL

Protein dish with steamed vegetables

Mid-Afternoon Snack – SUBSTITUTION METHOD

Two glasses of water

Wait at least ten minutes, and then eat strips of vegetables with some added herbs

Dinner – HWC MEAL

Vegetable soup and large mixed vegetable salad with nonfat dressing

Dessert: Unsweetened applesauce

You will notice that except for the fruit dessert, I do not mention eating a snack after dinner. We all know that it is better not to eat after dinner. This is true from both a weight loss and a digestive point of view. However, if you feel a strong craving, implement the Substitution method. Some people who suffer from cravings in the evening find that eating a small fruit dessert helps prevent these cravings.

CHAPTER 7
PHASE 2

PHASE 2 AT A GLANCE

For all the weeks in Phase 2,

Continue
- High-Water-Content (HWC) Meal once a day
- Substitution Method between meals
- Main One-Concentrated-Food (One CF) Meal for the main meal
- Light One-Concentrated-Food (One CF) Meal for the lighter meal

In Addition   Increase your cardiovascular exercise and add some strengthening exercises:

Weeks 1 and 2   Ten to fifteen minutes of cardiovascular exercise plus basic strengthening exercises, five times a week

Week 3   Fifteen to twenty minutes of cardiovascular exercise plus strengthening exercises, five times a week

THE ACCUMULATION PHASE

After five weeks of Phase 1, you will move on to Phase 2. Phase 2 lasts a minimum of three weeks.

During Phase 2, you will reinforce the subconscious traces that have been established during the previous Phase. It is generally accepted that about *thirty days* are needed before a new habit sets in and starts to become second nature.[1] Besides a slight increase in exercise, the weeks of Phase 2 are simply a continuation of the final week of Phase 1. Therefore, if you

---

1.   See Jerusalem Talmud, *Ta'anis* 1:1. See also *Shulchan Aruch, Orach Chaim* 114:8,9.

are already following a well-balanced exercise program (cardiovascular and strengthening exercises), Phase 2 will simply be a continuation of the final week of Phase 1. There will be no changes or additions. Only an inner change will take place, a subconscious accumulation of traces.

It is true that we are constantly reinforcing the accumulation of traces of our habits. However, during this stage, you will experience the most significant part of the Subconscious Accumulation Process. Weight loss accelerates and feelings of energy and health abound. In fact, most people lose five to ten pounds during Phase 2.

Phase 2 represents the ultimate eating program according to Rambam. This Phase is extremely effective in cleaning out your system. You will experience both a physical and psychological cleansing. Unhealthy cravings and bad eating habits will rapidly diminish. I know this may sound too good to be true, but *it works* – it really works!

It's not surprising that some people have continued with the guidelines of this Phase for the long term, even after having reached their goal weight. You can also choose to prolong this Phase for a longer period of time. Obviously, the longer you stay on this Phase, the more you will affect your personal subconscious accumulation process. However, it should be followed for a minimum of three weeks. Everyone is unique, so gauge what time period works best for *you*. Later, we will explain what signs to look for which will indicate that it is time to move on to Phase 3.

PHASE 2 / WEEK 1–WEEK 3

These are the only changes you will make during Phase 2:

Weeks 1 and 2 Ten to fifteen minutes of cardiovascular exercise plus basic strengthening exercises, five times a week

Week 3 Fifteen to twenty minutes of cardiovascular exercise plus strengthening exercises, five times a week

PACE OF EXERCISE

During Phase 2, you will increase the duration of your cardiovascular exercise. The correct pace and amount of this type of exercise is important at this stage.

The following hints have been included to help you achieve your optimum pace of exercise:

Rambam writes:

> Continue to exercise as long as your facial appearance is normal, the pace of exercise is being maintained, body warmth is stable and you are perspiring.[1]

A simple but useful measure is the "talk test." If you are doing moderate exercise, you should be able to have a normal conversation while doing it. If you are doing vigorous exercise you will usually find it hard to have a normal conversation. However, you should never be seriously out of breath.

---

1. *Medical Aphorisms* 18:14.

Modern-day fitness experts teach that in order to achieve the many benefits of exercise, you should maintain a certain level of exercise – called the "training zone" – during most of the workout. Amazingly, Rambam already makes mention of this concept: "One should begin exercising slowly, increasing [the pace] until he reaches the *optimum level* of exercise."[2]

What Is Your Training Zone?

The average person's resting pulse is 65 to 85 beats per minute.[3] When you exercise, your heart rate increases. Your training zone is a certain percentage of your maximum heart rate, which is calculated by taking the number 220 minus your age.

- For *moderate exercise*, your heart must beat at 50 to 70 percent of your maximum heart rate. Fifty percent is the lower end and 70 percent is the upper end.

- For *vigorous exercise*, your heart must beat at 70 to 85 percent of your maximum heart rate.[4]

EXAMPLE: FOR A THIRTY-YEAR-OLD:

Lower end for moderate exercise: $(220 - 30) \times 0.50 = 95$
Upper end for moderate exercise: $(220 - 30) \times 0.70 = 133$
Upper end for vigorous exercise: $(220 - 30) \times 0.85 = 161$

---

2. Ibid.
3. Note: Very fit people can have a slower resting pulse.
4. For more information, see the first Internet reference for Phase 2 in Appendix E (page 326).

AGE	MODERATE EXERCISE PULSE RATE	VIGOROUS EXERCISE PULSE RATE
20	100–140	140–170
30	95–133	133–161
40	90–126	126–153
50	85–119	119–144
60	80–112	112–136
70	75–105	105–127
80	70–98	98 –119

If you're just starting out on an exercise program, it is advisable to keep your heart rate at the lower end of your training zone.

How do you measure your heart rate? It's pretty simple. Just feel your pulse on your wrist or at the side of your windpipe, as soon as you stop exercising. Do not use your thumb to feel your pulse. To determine the number of heartbeats per minute, take your pulse for fifteen seconds and multiply by four. You must do it at this stage because the heartbeat slows down dramatically within the first minute after exercise.

The fitter you are, the harder you will have to work to reach your training zone. Bear in mind that there are also some people who have a natural faster heart rate, some who have a slower heart rate and others who have a heart rate which is artificially manipulated by medication. Still, for most people, the training zone equation is applicable, and it is a great way to monitor the level of your exercise workout. At the very minimum, it will add a bit of fun to your session, especially when you first begin an exercise program!

Always remember to drink enough water in order to avoid dehydration. The American Water Works Association recommends that a person drink water every twenty minutes when engaged in strenuous physical activity. This should be between a half and one cup of water every twenty minutes.

IS VIGOROUS EXERCISE BETTER?

The American College of Sports Medicine writes that for most people, exercising at the lower end of their training zone for a longer period of time may be better than exercising at the higher end of their training zone for a shorter period time.

After all is said and done, one of the most effective and convenient aerobic exercises is still a simple brisk walk for about thirty minutes. Walking outside in the fresh, crisp air enjoying the beautiful scenery will certainly add to the psychosomatic effect of the exercise. Furthermore, one study in the *Journal of the American Medical Association* shows that when it comes to losing weight, the difference between a thirty-minute-a-day moderate workout such as walking and a vigorous one-hour-a-day workout is only marginal.[5]

Now, this does not mean that you will not benefit from doing more exercise. The point is that you do not have to go crazy in order to experience the many benefits of exercising. In fact, too much exercise can actually be unhealthy for you and possibly even dangerous. It goes without saying that this applies to anyone who is not fit, but even if you are already fit, excessive exercise can still harm your health. Furthermore, if you are too extreme, it is likely that you will ultimately fail to do even that which is necessary. On this note Rambam writes:

5. Sora Song, "Exercise: What a Little Can Do," *Time*, September 22, 2003.

Not everyone can tolerate very vigorous exercise, nor is it necessary.[6]

Strenuous exercise dries out the body and makes it stiff, affecting sensation and slowing down the intellect.[7]

Elsewhere Galen sums it up:

The amount of exercise applicable in every individual case must be determined on an individual basis. *The right quality is of no use if the quantity is wrong.*[8]

THE STRENGTHENING INGREDIENT

During Phase 2, you will introduce some basic strengthening exercises to your exercise program. I will mention a few different options, including one that requires no equipment and can take as little as five minutes. Clear guidelines will be outlined.

Everyone seems to agree that cardiovascular exercise is the centerpiece of any exercise program. However, strengthening exercises are also an important part of a well-balanced program. Research has shown that basic strengthening exercises are safe and effective for men and women of all ages, including those who are not in perfect health.[9] In fact, people with health concerns – including heart disease or arthritis – often benefit the most from an exercise program that includes strengthening exercises a few times each week.

6. *Regimen of Health* 1:3.
7. *Medical Aphorisms* 18:9.
8. See *Galen: Selected Works*, pp. 299–304 (the exercise with the small ball).
9. For more information, see the second Internet reference for Phase 2 in Appendix E (page 326).

In addition, as mentioned earlier, Rambam and the ancient physicians also write about the importance of a well-balanced exercise program.[10]

Strengthening exercises build muscle mass and bone density. In addition, strength training has been shown to be especially effective in reducing the signs and symptoms of arthritis, osteoporosis and back pain. Moreover, strength training is important for weight control. How can this be?

Individuals who have more muscle mass have a higher metabolic rate. Muscle is active tissue which consumes calories. Strength training can cause up to a 15 percent increase in metabolic rate, which is enormously helpful for weight loss and long-term weight control.[11]

When strengthening exercises are done after the cardiovascular workout, they add further to the cardiovascular effect. However, you may find it more convenient to split your workout. You could do cardiovascular exercises in the morning and strengthening exercises at night. Some studies have shown that breaking up exercise sessions actually increases their overall effect.

You don't have to use weights to do strengthening exercises. In fact, one of the most effective ways to do them is by using the weight of your body. You can do these exercises in the convenience of your own home, or wherever else you may be. Both men and women, of all ages, can do them.

When performing strengthening exercises, it is important to concentrate on the three main muscle groups: the upper body, the stomach and the lower body. Relax: These exercises are very simple, and they shouldn't take much more than five minutes a day. Yet you will see amazing results and will enjoy a healthier body. You will be creating firm, healthy muscles. Just be sure to be consistent and give your body a chance to show these results.

10. See Phase 1, Week 2.
11. See the second Internet reference for Phase 2 in Appendix E (page 326).

These are the three basic groups of strengthening exercises:

1. **Lower body** – Starter Squats or regular Squats strengthen quadriceps (the greater extensor muscle of the front of the thigh), buttocks, hips, knees and back

2. **Stomach or abdominals** ("abs") – Upper and lower
   - Abs Crunches work the upper abdominals
   - Bent-Knee Raises or Leg Lifts work the lower abdominals

3. **Upper body** – Wall Push-Ups or conventional Push-Ups strengthen your arms, shoulders, and chest

Of course, there are many other types of basic strengthening exercises which can work all the different parts of your body. There are biceps, triceps, shoulder, back, leg, stomach and chest exercises. However, the exercises mentioned above will give you a basic workout for the body's main muscle groups. If you want, you can add light weights such as dumbbells or heavier weights such as a barbell or a bench press to your strengthening exercise routine.[12] In the Practical Method section below, I will explain how you can add these exercises to a basic workout depending on your level of fitness.

Obviously, a gym has the biggest variety of advanced strengthening exercise equipment, but you can buy reasonably priced basic equipment for home use. Today, most exercise equipment comes with short tutorials outlining basic strengthening exercises. For a more advanced personalized

---

12. When using weights, it is necessary to wait a day before performing that same strengthening exercise again, in order to allow that particular muscle to build up again. For example, if you do biceps exercises with weights one day, you can do leg exercises with weights the next day. But you should wait until the day after that before doing biceps exercises with weights again.

routine, you can peruse one of the myriad exercise books on the market or ask an exercise trainer.[13]

The benefits of adding some simple strengthening exercises to your program are immeasurable. It is the strengthening exercises in particular that will leave you feeling and looking your best.

I cannot stress enough: It is not the direct results of exercise that are as important as the overall commitment to a beneficial lifestyle that results from exercise. If you ever feel down about the way you are eating, get up and go to the gym or go do some exercise. I know it is hard, but after a rigorous workout you will feel energized and much more committed to get back or stay on track. This point is fundamental. After all, we are all human beings and no one is perfect. Exercise is one of the best motivational sources you will ever find!

13. The American College of Sports Medicine (ACSM) and American Council on Exercise (ACE) provide the most advanced and current scientific information regarding an exercise program for total fitness. If fulfilling their requirements is important to you, be sure your trainer is an ACE® – certified professional and/or familiar with ACSM guidelines.

PHASE 2 / WEEK 1–WEEK 3
PRACTICAL METHOD

During Phase 2, except for exercise, you will simply continue to reinforce the guidelines of the final week of Phase 1. You will probably never be hungry and yet you will still lose weight quickly. If you do feel hungry, check that you are actually following our guidelines. Don't try to stint yourself; it will backfire! Just stick to the guidelines of the Life-Transforming Diet.

However, this is how your exercise program will change:

WEEK 1

1. Increase your five to ten minutes of *cardiovascular exercise* to ten to fifteen minutes, five times a week.

2. Add some *strengthening exercises* to your exercise program, five times a week.

Continue this exercise routine during Week 2.

WEEK 3

1. Increase your *cardiovascular exercise* to fifteen to twenty minutes, five times a week.

2. If you are ready, add to or increase your *strengthening exercises*, i.e. go from the "very basic" option to the "basic" option, or from the "basic option" to the "basic plus" option (see below). Please see page 222 for an optional simple dumbbell program that can be done at home.

FROM THEORY TO PRACTICE

The following strengthening exercises do not require any equipment, and they can be done in the comfort of your home in a short amount of time. I have given you three basic strengthening exercise workout options. If you have not done any strengthening exercises before, you may want to start with the "very basic" option. If you are in better shape, you can begin with any of the options. Remember to build up slowly. You should be comfortable with your level of strengthening exercises before moving on to the next level.

On pages 184 through 187, you will find a detailed description of how to do these exercises. Of course, if you are already following a well-balanced exercise program, you can choose to continue with it.

For those of you who are unfamiliar with "exercise lingo," a *set* is a fixed amount of one exercise; a *repetition* is how many times you do that particular exercise in the set. For example, "Two sets of Starter Squats (10 repetitions)" means that you will be performing ten Starter Squats in a row (first set), then resting and performing another ten Starter Squats (second set).

Very Basic

- One set of Starter Squats using a chair or pillows (10–15 repetitions)

- Rest for about one minute and then do one set of Abs Crunches (10–15 repetitions)

- Rest for about one minute and then do one set of Wall Push-Ups (10–15 repetitions)

Basic

Replace the Starter Squats with regular Squats, and the Wall Push-Ups with conventional Push-Ups.

Basic Plus

You can do all three sets in a row; rest for one or two minutes and then repeat the three sets a second time. Also, in order to work both the upper and lower part of the abdomen, do Bent-Knee Raises or Leg Lifts for the second set. In other words:

First sets

- Begin with one set of regular Squats (10–15 repetitions)
- Then do one set of Abs Crunches (10–15 repetitions)
- Then do one set of conventional Push-Ups (10–15 repetitions)

After the first sets, rest for one or two minutes and then move on to the next sets.

Second sets

- Continue with one set of regular Squats (10–15 repetitions)
- Then do one set of Bent-Knee Raises or Leg-Lifts (10–15 repetitions)
- Then do one set of conventional Push-Ups (10–15 repetitions)

With all these exercises, you must remember to exhale while exerting yourself and inhale when returning to the starting position. Always remember to keep your stomach in during the duration of the exercise! (But don't forget to breathe.)

Squats

Regular Squat

- Stand with your feet slightly more than shoulder-width apart. Cross your arms over your chest.

- Lower yourself in a slow, controlled motion, buttocks out, until you reach a near-sitting position. Don't lower yourself too quickly, and make sure that your knees never come forward past your toes.

- Pause and then slowly rise back up to a standing position. Keep your knees over your ankles and your back straight.

If this exercise is too difficult, you can do *Starter Squats*: Put a chair in back of you. Sit down and then stand up, employing the same techniques stated above for regular Squats. If you are unable to go all the way down, place a couple of pillows on the chair or only squat down four to six inches. Remember to always keep your back straight.

Once you can do two sets of 10 to 15 repetitions, you can move on to the regular Squat without a chair, as explained above.

Sit-Ups

Abs Crunch – Upper Abs

- Lie on your back. Bend your knees, but keep both feet on the floor.

- Place your hands behind your head. This is simply for comfort; it is not an active part of this exercise. Don't pull on your neck with your hands.

- Slowly raise your shoulders and upper back off the floor. Exhale as you rise.

- Slowly lower your shoulders to the floor, just short of your head touching the floor. Inhale as you return to the starting position.

Bent-Knee Raise – Lower Abs

- Lie on your back and place both hands behind your head. Bend your knees at a 90 degree angle.

- Slowly raise both your legs. But keep your knees at that same angle. Your knees should not move at all. Exhale as you raise your legs.

- Slowly return to the starting position, just short of your feet touching the floor. Inhale as you lower your legs.

- Your back should remain against the floor throughout the whole exercise.

- Stop this exercise if any pain is felt in the back.

Some people may feel more comfortable with a similar but nevertheless different version of this exercise called the *Leg Lift*. With the Leg Lift, you do not start off with your knees bent at a 90 degree angle. Instead, keep your legs together on the floor, bending your knees only slightly, and then raise your legs off the ground. Pull your knees toward your chest until they form almost a 90 degree angle with the floor. (During this motion, your knees do not remain at the same angle at which they started, as they did with the Bent-Knee Raise.) Slowly return to the starting position, just short of your feet touching the floor.

Push-Ups

There are different variations of Push-Ups which work different parts of your chest.

Some people, often women, will want to start off with the Wall Push-Up.

This type of push-up works the middle chest.

Wall Push-Up

- Facing a wall, lean your body forward and place your hands against the wall at about shoulder height and shoulder-width apart.

- Bend your elbows as you lower your upper body toward the wall in a slow, controlled motion, keeping your feet planted on the ground.

- Pause for a moment and then slowly push yourself back until your arms are straight, with a slight bend in the elbows.

Once you can do two sets of 10 to 15 repetitions, you can move on to regular Push-Ups, which are done on the floor. Depending on how you position your hands and feet, this push-up works either your upper or your lower chest.

Regular Push-Up

- Lie on the floor face down with your chest touching the floor. Place your hands on either side of your shoulders.

- Your toes should be curled under and your feet hip-width apart. Raise your body until your arms are straight, with a slight bend in the elbows.

- Slowly lower your body, until you are about one inch above the ground, and then raise your body again.

Positioning your hands this way will work your upper chest. If you put your feet on a small bench, you will work your lower chest.

With all types of Push-Ups, be sure to keep your back straight – no sagging in the midsection of your body.

INSIGHTS AND SUCCESS STORIES

Deb from the United States lost 25 pounds – "worried friends"

I lost six pounds on Phase 1. I felt my eating and lifestyle habits slowly changing within me. Within three weeks on Phase 2, I lost another seven pounds. The weight loss was gaining momentum fast, and in a very short time, I had lost about fifteen pounds. What an exhilarating feeling! But it was much more than just a superficial experience. I was experiencing both an inner and an outer change. This really is a "life-transforming" diet. My family and close friends are so proud of me. Of course, there are some so-called "friends" who are "worried" about my weight loss: "It's enough already; be careful!" Maybe it's a bit of jealousy?

SUMMARY / PHASE 2

THE PHASE

Weeks 1 through 3

Continue the eating regimen from the final week of Phase 1

IN ADDITION…

Week 1

Increase cardiovascular exercise to ten to fifteen minutes, and *add* basic strengthening exercises, five times a week

Week 2

Reinforce the guidelines of Week 1

Week 3

Increase cardiovascular exercise to fifteen to twenty minutes, and *continue* with strengthening exercises, five times a week

DAILY REGIMEN

Meals

- High-Water-Content Meal
- Main One CF Meal
- Light One CF Meal

Between Meals

- Substitution Method – four preferences

Exercise

- Depending on the week, ten to twenty minutes of cardiovascular exercise, plus strengthening exercises, five times a week

A SAMPLE DAY IN PRACTICE

This is what your day could look like if you made breakfast your high-water-content meal and you did your exercise before breakfast:

Upon Awakening

Two glasses of water

Exercise – EXERCISE PROGRAM

Ten to twenty minutes of cardiovascular exercise and some strengthening exercises

Breakfast – HWC MEAL

Bowl of mixed fruit with a topping of nuts

Mid-Morning Snack – SUBSTITUTION METHOD

Two glasses of water

Iced drink and fruit

Lunch – LIGHT ONE CF MEAL

Tasty Tub version: salad with protein topping

Wait at least one to two hours after lunch and drink two glasses of water

Mid-Afternoon Snack – SUBSTITUTION METHOD

Two glasses of water

Nonfat yogurt

Strips of vegetables

Dinner – MAIN ONE CF MEAL

Baked flesh protein dish with steamed vegetables

CHAPTER 8
PHASE 3

For all the weeks in Phase 3,

Continue
- High-Water-Content (HWC) Meal once a day
- Fifteen to twenty minutes of cardiovascular exercise plus strengthening exercises, five times a week
- Substitution Method between meals
- Main One-Concentrated-Food (One CF) Meal OR Light One-Concentrated-Food (One CF) Meal once a day

In Addition You may have a Mixed Meal once a day and you will have more dessert options

THE INTEGRATION PHASE

Phase 3 is called the Integration Phase because in this Phase you will be able to eat any type of meal. You will not be limited to one concentrated food at all your meals. You can have one Mixed Meal a day. You will also have more dessert options.

Of course, by now, your new positive habits are subconsciously accumulating, so the meals you will want to eat, as well as your whole approach to eating in general, will be more sober than they were before you began the Life-Transforming Diet.

Some people may want to stay on Phase 2 for a longer period of time. Some even stay on Phase 2 until they are down to their goal weight, as progress is rapid and the vibrant feeling is exhilarating. Staying longer on Phase 2 will certainly add to your subconscious accumulation process. In fact, there are even people who have remained on Phase 2 for the long term, even after having reached their goal weight. Everyone is unique, so gauge what time period works best for YOU.

If you have chosen to prolong Phase 2, yet have started feeling that you want a greater variety of foods at a meal, this is most probably a sign that you should move on to Phase 3. Don't worry; you will definitely continue to lose weight at a very good pace during Phase 3 and beyond.

Remain on Phase 3 until you have reached your goal weight.

PHASE 3

Method	– Mixed Meal
	– More dessert options
Continue	– High-Water-Content (HWC) Meal once a day
	– Fifteen to twenty minutes of cardiovascular exercise plus strengthening exercises, five times a week
	– Substitution Method between meals
	– Main One-Concentrated-Food (One CF) Meal or Light One-Concentrated-Food (One CF) Meal once a day

MIXED MEAL

Many people get hooked on the One CF Meal. It's practical, enjoyable, and has many physiological advantages! But by now, you have regained better inner focus, and portion control has started to feel more natural. In today's world, some of us may find a One CF Meal a bit too restricting on a continual basis, and therefore the Mixed Meal presents a realistic alternative.

A Mixed Meal allows you to eat both types of concentrated foods at a meal. You can eat a meat or white cheese sandwich, chicken and potatoes, meatballs and pasta, or any starch with any protein at the same meal. Any meal which includes both protein and starches is considered a Mixed Meal.

Because of the variety of meal options available on the Life-Transforming Diet, you won't feel psychologically "strangled." You are empowered to cope with whatever situation presents itself, without "going off the diet."

TAKING SECONDS

Clearly, Rambam was not against eating more than one main concentrated food at a meal. In fact, he often discusses the sequence of foods to be eaten when different types of concentrated foods are eaten at the same meal.[1] He also writes, "A wise person eats only one *or two* foods at a meal, consuming enough to sustain himself."[2] Still, he believed that a meal containing only one concentrated food offers the optimum method for digestion and prevention of overeating. This is why we will continue to eat a One CF Meal once a day for the long term. But from Phase 3 and on, we have the option to eat one Mixed Meal a day.

But how can we eat a meal with more than one concentrated food and still prevent overeating? Take your normal portion of food, but take seconds only of the vegetables. It may also help to start the meal with a salad, vegetable entrée or soup. Then take only one helping of protein and starches. The essence of these measures is to avoid second helpings of concentrated foods. Taking seconds of vegetables is crucial when eating a Mixed Meal because you do not have the digestive and other advantages of the One CF Meal.

The digestive system requires much less energy to digest vegetables than it does to digest protein or starch. As a result, your body can deal far more effectively with larger amounts of vegetables than it can with concentrated foods. I have yet to meet someone who experiences that heavy, "sick" feeling after eating a few generous portions of salad or a vegetable dish. Furthermore, vegetables are high in fiber, which leaves you feeling full and not craving more. They are also low-calorie foods, as we have already learned. For all these reasons, it is very hard to overeat at a meal if you take extra portions of vegetables.

1. See *Mishneh Torah, Hilchos De'os* 4:7.
2. Ibid., 5:1.

In practice, if you were eating a dinner consisting of salmon, couscous and salad, then the portion of salmon and couscous would be limited to a single portion. If you still felt hungry, you would be able to continue with second or even third helpings of the salad. Second helpings of the concentrated foods would not be an option.

At first, this will take a bit of mind conditioning. Take a normal portion of food and say to yourself, "This is the amount of food I *want* and *need* to eat. If I eat any more food, it can only do me harm, physically and otherwise." Be honest: How often do you really enjoy a second helping after a mixed meal? Generally, when we take a second helping, we are eating with our eyes. How often do you walk away from a meal in which you took seconds, with feelings of guilt, disappointment and lethargy? Our Mixed Meal method guarantees that you will walk away from the meal satisfied, without feeling lethargic or "stuffed."

YOUR PERSONAL MEAL SCHEDULE

Through all the Phases and beyond, you always eat one High-Water-Content meal a day. But regarding the two main meals, from Phase 3 and on, you no longer have to eat two One CF Meals a day. For example, you could eat any kind of sandwich for lunch, such as a (low-fat or nonfat) white cheese sandwich or an egg sandwich, along with a vegetable side dish. This is of course a Mixed Meal, because you are eating starch and protein at the same meal. For dinner, you could eat your regular main meal such as chicken or fish with (non-starchy or medium-starchy) vegetables. This is a Main One CF Meal because you are eating only one concentrated food.

In general, I think it is best to make your heavier main meal a Main One CF Meal. The reason is that most people eat the biggest quantities at this meal.

The whole family may eat this meal together, and so it will often be drawn out. Unfortunately, this usually leads to overeating at this meal.

Furthermore, this meal often consists of larger amounts of protein, and protein takes longer to digest than starches. Thus, if you make your heavier meal a Mixed Meal instead of a Main One CF Meal, you will also have a starch side dish. This will stimulate your appetite further, making it even harder to control quantities. A Mixed Meal is also harder to digest. Making your heavier meal a One CF Meal will insure that it will be digested even more efficiently, and you can still take seconds of the protein. You are better off making your other, lighter main meal a Mixed Meal.

Also, many people prefer to eat grains with dairy – such as hot cereal with milk, or grains with protein – such as a white cheese, meat or tuna sandwich. In these Mixed Meal cases, you are eating smaller quantities of protein or lighter proteins. Moreover, this is usually a quicker meal, and the amounts of food are easier to digest. The Mixed Meal guidelines will insure that you will not overeat at this lighter main meal.

However, if you choose to eat a Mixed Meal for your larger main meal, such as meat and potatoes, meatballs with pasta or fish and rice, I suggest that you make your lighter main meal that day a Light One CF Meal instead of a Main One CF meal. Your body will be better prepared to digest that larger Mixed Meal.

These are only suggestions; ultimately it is your choice. See what works best for you. The Sample Day in Practice at the end of this chapter (pages 209 through 211) will show you how a Mixed Meal can add a lot of flexibility to your meal choices.

Remember: You should never eat more than one Mixed Meal a day, and you should always eat one HWC meal a day.

HELPFUL HINTS

If you still feel hungry after eating your meal, then leave the table and wait five to ten minutes. Many times, my wife would catch me hanging around the food pantry after finishing a meal. "Sit down and wait for a few minutes," she would suggest. I would sit down begrudgingly, knowing all too well that within a few minutes I would no longer crave a treat. You don't start feeling satisfied from a meal immediately after you finish it. Moreover, the urge to eat more could simply be a post-meal bad habit to which you have become accustomed.

At first, you may find it helpful to brush your teeth right after the meal. Doing so after dinner is especially effective. Also, try not to prepare more food than you actually need so you will not be tempted to have seconds and thirds. But even if you do cook in bulk, don't put food platters on the table – except for salads and vegetable dishes. Serve yourself from the stove (or in the kitchen if you're eating in the dining room), and put the extra food away before you start to eat. For those who have the bad habit of eating everyone's leftovers, get someone else to clear the table.

MORE DESSERT OPTIONS

At this stage, you are in a position to be more liberal with your dessert options. In fact, Rambam was not against taking "a little" bit of sweets after the meal.[3] But please do not take this out of context. Rambam says to take "a little," and you have to be at the stage where you can keep it to "a little." Honestly, it would be better to wait until you are down to your goal weight before starting with this – not because these options are very fattening or very unhealthy, but because initially we are trying to cleanse our bodies

3. *Regimen of Health* 1:13.

and remove unhealthy cravings. That is why we allow only applesauce and certain types of fruit for the dessert option during Phases 1 and 2.

On the other hand, some people may want a greater variety of dessert options by Phase 3, and they may not want to wait until they reach their goal weight. After all, it could take some people six months to a year to reach goal. For them, the risks are too high not to offer more dessert options, because it could possibly jeopardize their whole eating plan.

So if you are in the mood for something sweet besides fruit or if you are faced with a very fattening and unhealthy dessert and you really want to indulge, the following desserts are much better options and the best choice at this stage. They can satisfy any sweet tooth. In effect, you are indulging an unhealthy craving with smarter choices.

In addition to the dessert fruits we mentioned in Phase 1, Rambam also suggests having pistachios or almonds at the end of the meal.[4] Sorbet or gelatin desserts are low-calorie, refreshing dessert options. Non-dairy ices or sugar-free Tofutti pops are great because they are extremely low in calories and it is very easy to control quantity. Nonfat frozen yogurt or nonfat ice cream are also options. Hard candies can also be very effective in satisfying a craving for dessert. They take time to consume and are usually very low in calories.

So until you reach your goal weight, these are your dessert options during Phase 3, in their order of preference:

- Ice pops, sugar-free (each has 0 fat, 15–25 calories/62–104 klj)

- Ice pops, sugar (each has 0 fat, 40–90 calories/188–376 klj)

- Tofutti pops, non-dairy, sugar-free (each has 0 fat, 30 calories/125 klj)

---

4. *Treatise on Asthma* 3:10.

- Gelatin dessert, sugar-free (½ cup has 0 fat, 10 calories/42 klj)

- Hard candies, sugar-free (1 piece has 0 fat, 5–10 calories/20–41 klj)

- Hard candies, sugar (1 piece has 0 fat, 10–24 calories/41–100 klj)

- Sorbet, nonfat, sugar (½ cup has 0 fat, 80 calories/335 klj)

- Gelatin dessert, sugar (½ cup has 0 fat, 80 calories/335 klj)

- Pistachios, 20 nuts (7 grams of fat, 80 calories/335 klj)

- Almonds, 13 medium (7.5 grams of fat, 85 calories/355 klj)

- Frozen yogurt, nonfat (½ cup has 0 fat, 90 calories/377 klj)

- Ice cream, soft-serve, nonfat (½ cup has 0 fat, 90 calories/377 klj)

As you can see, 90 calories' worth of some of these desserts is a large quantity: 3–6 sugar-free ice pops, 3 sugar-free Tofutti pops, 4½ cups of a sugar-free gelatin dessert and 9–18 sugar-free hard candies. I am certainly not suggesting that you eat the maximum quantity of low-calorie foods! However, it makes an important psychological point. Sometimes, we are not aware that certain high-calorie foods come with a steep caloric price relative to how much we can eat. You could be eating much better foods and in larger quantities, certainly from a weight-loss perspective.

I am aware that the sugar-free options will cause some eyebrows to be raised. As I have mentioned, artificial sweeteners are a subject of debate among the health professionals. Certainly, natural products are preferable, and there are certain foods which are low enough in calories such as regular nonfat ice pops. However, when it comes to soda or certain desserts, there is a big difference between the regular and diet versions. If you choose to eat these foods, the low-calorie items are preferable from a weight loss perspective. Everyone agrees that being overweight or obese is extremely dangerous, and we are focusing on reducing that danger. Once you are down to your correct weight, you can choose to start zoning in to potential health issues that are not weight issues. Nevertheless, if you feel strongly about avoiding these products, stick to the *regular* low-calorie items or simply avoid those dessert choices altogether.

The mention of calories does not mean that you should become obsessed or feel trapped with calorie counting. As I mentioned, calories only become applicable when comparing non-nutritious foods (or when limiting quantities between meals). The point here is that it is very hard to limit quantities of dessert. The above choices, which range from 0 to 90 calories, simply insure that you will not overeat a dessert or choose high-fat desserts.

Various brands of the dessert options mentioned above differ in their calories per serving. Some are higher than our guidelines. However, there are many brands which fit into these guidelines. So pay attention to the nutrition label on the package. We will discuss reading nutrition labels in Chapter 13.

Take note: Everyone reacts differently to food choices at different stages, so gauge your own reaction honestly. If after eating one of these dessert options, you find that you are craving more between meals, or if you are finding it hard to limit the quantities, then keep these options to a minimum. In fact, I suggest that until you are close to your goal weight, you should enjoy these dessert options only on special occasions or when you are faced with a much worse dessert choice. You do not want to embolden any unhealthy cravings.

Stay focused! We all know that it is not "hunger" that we experience at the end of a meal. After all, we have just finished eating! We are simply satisfying our sweet tooth, and this does not require large quantities. In fact, for many people, it is mostly about knowing that other dessert options exist. These dessert options give you the tools and knowledge to deal with a craving at the end of a meal – but only you can know whether it is worthwhile to implement or whether it will backfire and set off a cycle of giving in to unhealthy cravings.

Remember, these are not food options between the meals. You are not ready to eat other foods besides the four preferences of the Substitution Method until you are down to your goal weight *and* your inner controls are in better focus. At that stage, you will be able to eat these foods as snacks between meals and you will also have the option to eat other, higher calorie desserts. This will be discussed in the next chapter.

EXERCISE

By now, you are following a basic, well-balanced exercise program. If you would like to step it up a notch – and you feel you are ready – you can move both your cardiovascular and your strengthening exercises up to the next level.

Regarding cardiovascular exercise: According to The National Center for Chronic Disease Prevention and Health Promotion, in order to achieve all the benefits from exercising, an adult should do:

— Moderate exercise for [at least] thirty minutes, five or more times week,

OR

— Vigorous exercise for [at least] twenty minutes, three or more times a week.[5]

5.   For more information, see the first Internet reference for Phase 3 in Appendix E (page 326).

The following are examples of moderate and vigorous exercise:[6]

MODERATE	VIGOROUS
Walking briskly	Race walking, jogging or running
Golf, pulling or carrying clubs	Swimming laps
Recreational swimming	Mowing the lawn with a hand mower
Mowing the lawn with a power motor	Tennis singles
Tennis doubles	Bicycling more than 10 mph, or on steep uphill terrain
Bicycling 5 to 9 mph, level terrain, or with a few hills	Moving or pushing furniture
Scrubbing floors or washing windows	Circuit training
Weight lifting, Nautilus machines or free weights	

In Chapter 7, I mentioned how you can measure the pace of your exercise with the "training zone." Your heart rate during exercise can be an even more precise way to measure whether an exercise is moderate or vigorous.

Regarding strengthening exercises, you could simply add more repetitions to each set. For example, you could do two sets of 30 Abs Crunches

6. For more information, see the second Internet reference for Phase 3 in Appendix E (page 326).

instead of 10 to 15 repetitions. Another option is to keep the same amount of repetitions but to do three sets instead of two. If you want to add a greater variety of strengthening exercises, there are biceps, triceps, shoulders, back, leg and chest exercises. As I already mentioned, a more advanced option is to add light weights such as dumbbells or heavier weights such as a barbell or a bench press to your strengthening exercise routine. A gym offers a large selection of more advanced equipment, but there are many machines available on the market for home use.

Let me stress that you must comfortably be able to do the fifteen to twenty minutes of cardiovascular exercise along with the strengthening exercises five times a week (introduced at the end of Phase 2), before even thinking about increasing your exercise load. You can only build from a solid foundation. There are really so many different options when it comes to exercise. But the key is to keep it simple and practical.

Often, it is easier to be motivated about exercise when you have a clearly defined goal, as you have during weight loss. This is especially crucial the closer you get to goal weight, because then the temptation to become lax about exercising increases. It is important to renew your enthusiasm, because exercise is a cornerstone in the preservation of health, regardless of your weight.

I have found that it is effective to compartmentalize your exercise program in your head. Choose three non-consecutive days, such as Sunday, Tuesday and Thursday, as the foundation of your exercise program. (Remember, you need a one-day rest between the same weight-strengthening exercises.) From this base, add two other days a week of a different, perhaps lighter, type of exercise. This way your exercise program seems less daunting and easier to accept.

SUPPORT SYSTEM

You will continue on Phase 3 until you have reached your goal weight. In fact, you will continue to apply its main principles for the long term. Speaking of which, one of the latest diet surveys shows that although few dieters have long-term success, those who have maintained their weight loss attribute much of their success to support groups. We cannot underestimate the encouragement and help that come from a support system. We all thrive on love, friendship and encouragement. Moreover, we are profoundly influenced by our immediate surroundings.

As Rambam writes:

> It is the nature of a person's perceptions and actions to be influenced by his friends and associates.[7]

You will probably experience different reactions from people as you transform your eating habits. Some will encourage you, expressing full faith in your success. Others, whose verbal or non-verbal negativity probably stems from their own insecurities, will drain your enthusiasm. Other times you will find yourself in a situation where someone who may not intend to be unkind, will make you feel uncomfortable. For example, if you are a guest at a meal, the hostess might put you in a position where you feel obligated to eat all the different foods that are served. Similarly, you might be offered food by someone you wish to please, such as your mother, your grandmother or your mother-in-law. Sometimes, a spouse or family member may stock up the pantry and fridge with "delicacies," without realizing that it presents formidable challenges and temptations for you.

Situations such as those mentioned above make the lifestyle of the health-conscious or weight-conscious person a challenge to maintain. Therefore, it is imperative to remember that ultimately, your success hinges on your

---

7. See *Mishneh Torah, Hilchos De'os* 6:1.

maintaining responsibility for yourself and for your commitment to do what is best for you. *Make a commitment to yourself.* The key is knowing that you can always choose how you will respond to any situation.

A support system can really enhance the experience of this program. After all, we are all participants in at least one of the battles: to lose weight, to maintain weight or just to be health-conscious. Try to find a family member or a friend who is interested in learning and keeping our principles.

We are currently working on some exciting ideas for setting up Support Groups throughout the world. There are also some interesting possibilities for qualifying Support Group Leaders. Please stay in contact with us. (See Chapter 12, footnote 11, for our contact information.)

When you have established the positive habits of the Life-Transforming Diet, it is a good idea to teach the principles you have learned and implemented to someone who is interested in finding out more about this topic. It will add some fun to the process and it will make you feel committed to the program. You will read more intently and deeply when you know that you may have to teach some of the material to someone else. When you verbalize information to another interested person, it necessitates clarity of thought and expression on your part. You cannot fool yourself!

Remember, you are not alone! Others have felt similar yearnings, similar frustrations, similar disappointments and similar determinations. There is great joy and relief in that realization!

Yes, we are all travelers on the same journey to the same destination of "a healthy mind in a healthy body."

PHASE 3
PRACTICAL METHOD

If, after Phase 2, you begin to want a greater variety of food choices, go ahead and introduce a Mixed Meal into your meal schedule. At a Mixed Meal, you can eat a wider range of different foods and food groups, such as a protein sandwich or any protein main dish with any starch side dish.

At a Mixed Meal, take seconds only of non-starchy or medium-starchy vegetables. In other words, you should not have seconds of the concentrated foods. This is crucial, because a Mixed Meal does not have the digestive and other physiological advantages of a One CF Meal.

Starting off the meal with a vegetable entrée or soup is also a good idea. Then take only one helping of protein and carbohydrates.

You don't have to eat a Mixed meal every day. In the beginning of Phase 3, you may choose to eat a Mixed Meal a few times a week. But you no longer have to eat two One CF Meals every day.

This is my suggestion regarding your meals:

- Lightest meal: HWC Meal

- Heavier main meal: Main One CF Meal

- Lighter main meal: Mixed Meal

OR

- Lightest meal: HWC Meal

- Heavier main meal: Mixed Meal

- Lighter main meal: Light One CF Meal

Ultimately, your meal schedule is your choice, but you should never have more than one Mixed Meal a day, and you should always eat one HWC meal a day.

In Phase 3, you may also be more liberal with your dessert options. If you are in the mood for something sweet besides the dessert fruits listed in Phase 1, or if you are faced with a fattening and unhealthy dessert and want a more "dessert-like" alternative than the fruit, you may choose from the low-calorie dessert options listed on pages 198 through 199. They are good substitutes, and they will satisfy any craving you might have at the end of a meal.

If, after eating one of these dessert options, you find that you are craving more between meals, or if you are finding it hard to limit the quantities, then keep these options to a minimum or enjoy them only on special occasions.

By this stage, you are following a basic, well-balanced exercise program. If you feel at this point that you are ready to step it up a notch, you can advance both your cardiovascular and your strengthening exercises as explained above.

In Phase 1, Week 1, I mentioned that after Phase 2 you can change the position of your High-Water-Content Meal. For example, if you were eating a High-Water-Content Meal for breakfast during Phases 1 and 2, you can now switch it to lunch or dinner. It is up to you! (It's always best to try to stick to the same schedule so that a habit can be reinforced.)

Stay on Phase 3 until you reach your desired weight. A support system will enhance the experience of this program and assist you in achieving your long-term goals.

INSIGHTS AND SUCCESS STORIES

Zehava from South Africa – an answer to her prayers

A good friend of mine went on the Life-Transforming Diet and lost a ton of weight. In one night I read The Life-Transforming Diet, *and my life was transformed. After losing and regaining thousands of pounds, I finally found an answer to my prayers: a way of life that was healthy, spiritual, fulfilling, and that facilitates weight loss. I lost twenty pounds and my family loves my new look. Now, every time I reach for something I shouldn't, my seven-year-old asks if the Rambam allows it and the rest of the family makes sure I don't eat it.*

The age-old wisdom of the Rambam combined with David Zulberg's genius adaptation has provided me with a guide to enriching the quality of my life. With a ways to go and a lifetime of maintenance, I know my journey hasn't ended... but I feel confident that I have found a program that can help me to fulfill my potential and enable me to live my life feeling in control, in shape and inspired.

Miriam from the United States – gained weight and optimum health

Since I can remember, I had skimped on my food intake. I always felt the pressure to look "picture-perfect." Though never spoken about openly, this attitude is an accepted norm among my friends. As a result, I was not eating enough and I never even realized that I was underweight.

The Life-Transforming Diet has done just that – transformed my life. I am now eating regular nutritious meals and I enjoy my food without feeling guilty. Sometimes I still have to battle against old attitudes – especially when I'm under pressure – but now I have the tools to deal with myself and my thought patterns. I have gained some weight and I am much fitter than I ever remember being. I like the way I feel. I am much calmer. I can eat the way I want according to the guidelines of the program. I feel confident that I will not get fat, and I am ecstatic with how I look these days! My family and friends are very proud of me, and some of them have started the program as well.

SUMMARY / PHASE 3

THE PHASE

Option to substitute a Mixed Meal for a One CF Meal, once a day –
take seconds of vegetables only

DAILY REGIMEN

Meals

- High-Water-Content Meal
- Choose two: Light One CF Meal, Main One CF Meal, Mixed Meal
- Low-calorie dessert option

Between Meals

- Substitution Method – four preferences

Exercise

- If you are ready and if you want to, you may increase your
  cardiovascular and strengthening exercises.

A SAMPLE DAY IN PRACTICE

**If you make lunch your Mixed Meal and dinner a Main One CF Meal,
and you exercise between lunch and dinner:**

Upon Awakening

Two glasses of water

Breakfast – HWC MEAL

Bowl of mixed fruit

Mid-Morning Snack – SUBSTITUTION METHOD

Two glasses of water

Hot drink and yogurt

Lunch – MIXED MEAL

Any protein and salad in a pita

Take seconds of salad

Exercise – EXERCISE PROGRAM

Wait at least two hours after lunch and do fifteen to twenty minutes of cardiovascular exercise, plus strengthening exercises

Two glasses of water

Mid-Afternoon Snack – SUBSTITUTION METHOD

A little dried fruit

Dinner – MAIN ONE CF MEAL

Flesh protein and vegetable side dishes

Dessert: Sugar-free gelatin dessert

If you make dinner your Mixed Meal and breakfast a Light One CF Meal, and you exercise before breakfast:

Upon Awakening

Two glasses of water

Exercise – EXERCISE PROGRAM

Fifteen to twenty minutes of cardiovascular exercise, plus strengthening exercises

Breakfast – LIGHT ONE CF MEAL

Light Protein version: Vegetable omelet with salad

Mid-Morning Snack – SUBSTITUTION METHOD

Two glasses of water

Hot drink and fruit

Lunch – HWC MEAL

Large chef's salad with fat-free dressing and a baked butternut squash, OR a bowl of mixed fruit with a topping of nuts

Mid-Afternoon Snack – SUBSTITUTION METHOD

Two glasses of water

½ cup of low-fat cottage cheese and strips of vegetables

Dinner – MIXED MEAL

Grilled protein dish with potatoes or rice and an optional small glass of unsweetened wine

Dessert: two ice pops

I have given you the principles through which you can achieve health and permanent weight loss. Now, you adapt them to suit you and your lifestyle. You need no longer be a victim of food. You can choose what to eat and when to eat it, according to the principles of the Life-Transforming Diet.

CHAPTER 9
DAILY CALORIE REQUIREMENTS

A WELL-BALANCED DIET

The principles of the Life-Transforming Diet are in alignment with the recommendations of the most current United States Dietary Guidelines.[1] The Guidelines provide advice based upon scientific research to promote health and reduce risk of chronic diseases through diet and physical activity. Each food group provides a wide array of nutrients, so it is important to include all food groups in your daily diet: fruits, vegetables, grains, proteins, milk and healthy fats.

WILL EATING TOO FEW CALORIES AID WEIGHT LOSS?

Eating too few calories can actually stall weight loss. Your metabolism, which is the rate at which your body burns calories, slows down as a defense mechanism against starvation. In other words, deficient calorie intake puts the body into emergency mode and as a result starts hoarding

---

1. The Dietary Guidelines form the basis of Federal nutrition policy, education, and food assistance programs. By law (Public Law 101-445, Title III, 7 U.S.C. 5301 et seq.), the Dietary Guidelines are reviewed, updated if necessary, and published every five years. The process to create the Dietary Guidelines is a joint effort of the U.S. Department of Health and Human Services (HHS) and the U.S. Department of Agriculture (USDA).

calories by slowing down your metabolism. So even though you're eating fewer calories, your body may become incapable of losing weight, despite your efforts.

Eating too many calories also stalls weight loss, even if you are eating nutritious foods. Rambam makes it clear that overeating even the best foods is unhealthy. Excess intake of calories will lead to excess fat storage.

Calorie counting is not the main focus of the Life-Transforming Diet, because our main aim is to reinstate the integrity of our body's hunger and satiation signals. We accomplish this through a balance of nutritional, fitness and behavior modification principles. Obsession with calorie counting can lead to unhealthy eating habits, and perhaps also to a diet of nutritionally low-quality foods. Nonetheless, knowledge of calorie content can still be very useful and, if used appropriately, a very powerful tool to enhance our principles.

CALCULATING YOUR DAILY CALORIES

Weight management depends on the amount of energy you put into your body (food calories) versus the amount of energy you expend (activity). How do you know how many calories your body needs in order to reach or maintain a certain weight? By understanding your body's energy requirements.

There are three primary components that make up your body's energy expenditure: basal metabolic rate, energy expended during physical activity, and the thermic effect of food.

1. **Basal Metabolic Rate (BMR):** Most of the body's energy, about 60 to 70 percent in fact, goes to supporting the ongoing metabolic work of

the body's cells. This includes activities such as heartbeat, respiration and maintaining body temperature.

2. **Energy Expended During Physical Activity:** The second component of the equation depends upon your level of physical activity. Physical activity has a profound effect on human energy expenditure, and contributes 20 to 30 percent to the body's total energy output.

3. **Thermic Effect of Food:** The last component to calculate has to do with your body's management of food. Ten percent of the body's energy is required to digest food. This is referred to as the thermic effect of food (TEF).

Before we jump into equations it is important to know the minimum daily calorie requirements, no matter what you determine as your final personal calculation.

MINIMUM DAILY CALORIE REQUIREMENTS

– According to the National Institutes of Health, women should not consume less than 1,200 calories a day. Men shouldn't consume less than 1,500 calories a day.

– According to the Mayo Clinic, women who are between 250 and 300 pounds should consume no less than 1,400 calories per day, and men in that same category should consume no less than 1,600 calories per day.

Now let us look at some calculations, starting from simple to more complicated.

WEIGHT + ACTIVITY FORMULA

You can use this easy formula, which is a favorite of cardiologist Dr. Thomas Lee, editor-in-chief of the *Harvard Heart Letter*. It is for adults only.

1. Find your activity level (see below).

2. Multiply your current weight by the number indicated.

3. The result is the number of calories you need to maintain your weight.

4. Subtract 250 or 500 calories for weight loss. (250 calories for a half-pound weight loss per week and 500 calories for a one-pound weight loss per week.)

In other words, your current weight x activity level = weight maintenance, minus 250–500 calories for weight loss.

ACTIVITY LEVEL:

1) I almost never exercise:
   multiply your current weight by 12

2) I exercise lightly, 1 to 3 days a week:
   multiply your current weight by 13.5

3) I exercise moderately, 3 to 5 days a week:
   multiply your current weight by 15.5

4) I exercise vigorously, 6 to 7 days a week:
   multiply your current weight by 17

So for example: Let's say you weigh 135 pounds and do light exercise one to three days a week. Multiply 135 by 13.5 to get approximately 1,800 calories.

This is the number of calories you need to maintain your weight as it is. If you want to lose weight, try cutting out at least 250 calories a day, says Dr. Lee. In a year, if you make no other changes, you could be 26 pounds lighter. If you subtracted 500 calories a day you would lose one pound a week, which is about 52 pounds in a year. Exercise more and you could lose more.

MIFFLIN-ST. JEOR EQUATION

The ADA (American Dietetic Association) found the Mifflin-St. Jeor Equation to be the most accurate method. This is the one recommended by most nutrition professionals.

As you will soon see, this equation is quite involved, but we offer an online calculator that makes it a snap. You just enter your personal information and the calculator does all the converting and final results. This is how it is calculated if you want to do it alone:

Step 1: Take measurements of your weight and height, in order to obtain an accurate BMR. (Use a calculator to convert pounds to kilograms by dividing pounds by 2.2, and convert inches into centimeters by multiplying inches by 2.54.)

Step 2: Take these two numbers and plug them in to the Mifflin-St. Jeor Equation.

Males: BMR =
(10 x weight in kg) + (6.25 x height in cm) − (5 x age in years) + 5

Females: BMR =
(10 x weight in kg) + (6.25 x height in cm) − (5 x age in years) − 161

Step 3: Multiply the BMR obtained by the factor that best represents your level of activity.

- Sedentary (little to no activity): BMR x 1.2
- Light activity (exercise 1–3 days per week): BMR x 1.375
- Moderately active (exercise 3–5 days per week) BMR x 1.55
- Very active (exercise 6–7 days per week) BMR x 1.725
- Extremely Active (exercise twice a day) BMR x 1.9

The results obtained represent the total daily energy expenditure in calories needed to sustain your current body weight. Subtract the amount of calories per day (i.e., 250–500 calories) from the results in order to lose weight.

CONCLUSION

Comparing the results from the above two methods, for a female (let's call her Rachel) who weighs 135 pounds and is 5 ft 3 in, 31 years old, and doing light exercise one to three days a week:

- **Weight + Activity Method** = 1,822.5 calories
- **Mifflin-St. Jeor Equation** = 1,783 calories

These numbers are the calories this woman would need per day to maintain her current weight. She would then subtract 500 calories per day for a weight loss of one pound a week, which would give her between 1,283 and 1,500 calories per day. These numbers are still higher than the minimum daily calorie requirements mentioned above.

APPLYING DAILY CALORIE REQUIREMENTS TO THE LIFE-TRANSFORMING DIET

It is really quite simple to apply your daily calorie requirements to our principles. The Light/HWC meal has approximately 250 calories, and between-meal allowances are approximately 250 calories (120 calories of low-fat dairy twice a day, or low-fat dairy once a day and a Low-Cal Exception, or three fruits a day between meals). This gives you a total of 500 calories and leaves you with the One CF meal and the Mixed meal for the remainder of your total daily calorie allowance.

Step 1: Use one of the two daily calorie requirement formula methods mentioned above. Always make sure you do not go below the minimum daily requirement of 1,200 calories for women and 1,500 for men.

Step 2: Take your total and subtract 250–500 calories for weight loss, and another 500 calories to cover the Light meal and the Substitution method. The remaining number is the calorie allowance for the One CF meal and the Mixed meal, combined. You may divide your total between these two main meals as you see fit.

To use the same example above, i.e., for a female like Rachel:

- **Weight + Activity Method:** 1,822.5 calories (weight maintenance) minus 1,000 calories (500 for weight loss and 500 for the Light meal and the Substitution method) = **822.5** total calorie allowance for the One CF meal and the Mixed meal.
- **Mifflin-St. Jeor Equation:** 1,783 calories (weight maintenance) minus 1,000 calories (500 for weight loss and 500 for the Light meal and the Substitution method) = **783** total calorie allowance for the One CF meal and the Mixed meal.

If this particular female was aiming for a half-pound weekly weight loss with a goal of a 26-pound weight loss per year, her One CF and Mixed meals total calorie allowance would increase by 250 calories.

Technically, you could split the calorie allowance differently between the One CF and Mixed meals. For instance, you may choose to eat a larger One CF meal one day. In this case, you would make your Mixed meal a smaller meal. So if you have 1,000 calories *total* allowance for the One CF and the Mixed meal, you could have 300 calories at your Mixed meal and 700 calories at your One CF meal. We suggest you try keeping your meals somewhat balanced, as shown above, but you may customize your own meal preferences. We believe your largest meal of the day should be a One CF meal because it has the best digestive and weight loss results.

> REMEMBER: When you are at goal weight and no longer aiming for weight loss but weight maintenance, you could add back the 250–500 calories a day which you subtracted for weight loss. Exercise more, and you can add even more calories a day. These added calories should be added to your One CF meal and Mixed meal allowances, as the Light meal and Substitution method should preferably always remain constant at a combined total of approximately 500 calories.

No one is the same and it is hard to generalize when defining nutritional and daily requirements. In the long term, you will learn to customize your own particular schedule and lifestyle habits according to your personal goals.

Although calorie calculations are not actually required on the Life-Transforming Diet, they can enhance the program. They are especially useful if you experience a weight loss plateau. Sometimes calculating your daily calorie requirements will ensure that you are not actually overeating.

Most nutritionists will take calorie requirements into account. We have now provided *you* with these tools in order to help you succeed on your personal journey on the Life-Transforming Diet.

CHAPTER 10
SOME LT DIET UPDATES

HWC (HIGH-WATER-CONTENT) MEAL

Rambam writes that the number of meals eaten per day is of primary importance for maintaining health. He says that one should eat two meals a day:

> People have different habits regarding when they eat. Most of them eat in the morning and evening.[1]

The High-Water-Content meal is the perfect solution for our third "non-main meal" because it is low in calories, nutritious and has many digestive advantages.

Originally, there were only two options for the HWC meal on the Life-Transforming Diet. The first is a bowl of fruit or mixed fruit platter. (A small topping of nuts may be added.) The second is a salad with a nonfat, low-fat or homemade dressing. (Some people like to start with a vegetable soup. Medium-starchy vegetables such as carrots, butternut squash, pumpkin or beets may also be eaten with this vegetable meal. (A small topping of seeds may be added.)

Now there is a third option. The third option is any meal less than 250 calories (the "Light meal"). For example, you could have one and a half cups of Special K or any whole bran cereal (180 calories) with half a cup of nonfat/low-fat milk (30–50 calories). Another example is 2–3 slices of

---

1. *Treatise on Asthma* 6:1.

whole wheat bread (60–70 calories per slice) with nonfat or low-fat cream cheese and a side of vegetables. Two fried eggs with feta cheese or two fried eggs with one slice of toast (180 calories) is acceptable as well.

The logic is that a meal less than 250 calories is still considered within the parameters of a "non-main meal," which is the main goal of a high-water-content meal. That said, we still suggest that you try the fruit or vegetable option for at least the first week on the program, preferably for the whole of Phase 1. Only choose the Light meal option if you find it difficult to have fruits and vegetables. The reason for this is that fruits and vegetables will have an amazing cleansing effect on your system and it will also get you into the habit of including more of these crucial foods in your diet. Three small apples are about 250 calories. Assorted fruit will generally range between 150–250 calories and a plain salad with low-fat dressing is about 250 calories. After Phase 1, you can switch more freely between the three options.

The Light meal choice can also be a good opportunity to add more healthy grains to your diet. Some people may find this option more satisfying than the fruit or vegetable option in the long term. See the end of this chapter for two sample days with the Light meal option.

EXERCISE

Though not required, a dumbbell program will deliver terrific results and it can be done at home with very basic equipment. You can introduce dumbbell exercises during Phase 2. Remember to exhale during the exertion part of the exercise, and make sure that you are not experiencing back pain during any stage of the exercise. A minimum weight-training program according to the American College of Sports Medicine involves eight to ten different exercises. It is important to select at least one exercise for each major muscle group to ensure comprehensive muscle development. Exercise specialists agree that the following eight-move routine represents a basic, full-body exercise program for all levels. (Dumbbell exercises should be added to your routine only if you are comfortably doing the body strengthening exercises that we have already described in this book.)

1. Squat: Works your legs (buttocks to calves)

2. Lunge: Works your legs (buttocks to calves)

3. Bench press: Works your chest, shoulders and triceps

4. One arm row: Works your upper and lower back

5. Seated shoulder press: Works your shoulders

6. Seated triceps extension: Works your triceps

7. Biceps curl: Works your biceps

8. Crunch or Bicycle crunch: Works your abdominals

You can go to www.lifetransformingdiet.com for a description of these exercises. We suggest you begin with one set of 8 repetitions for each of the 8 different exercises, once or twice a week. When you are comfortable you can increase it to two sets, and then three sets. When you are comfortable with three sets, increase the frequency to two and then three or four times a week. If you want to see results, your minimum should eventually be two sets of the 8-move routine, twice a week.

WEIGHT-TRAINING GUIDELINES

Exercise Sequence: Start with the larger muscle groups so that you perform the most demanding exercises when you are the least fatigued. Another option is to group exercises into upper and lower body movements and to do only one type each day, as this provides recovery between exercises and decreases duration of the workout.

Exercise Duration: Training recommendation is 1–2 seconds for each lifting movement and 3–4 seconds for each lowering movement.

Exercise Interval: Rest 1–3 minutes between sets.

Exercise Resistance and Repetitions: 70–80 percent of maximum resistance is a sound training recommendation for safe and productive strength development (usually about 8–12 repetitions). One hundred percent represents the maximum amount of weight that you can lift just one time, usually while performing a leg press or bench press exercise. Lifting maximum weight loads is not recommended for most people because the risk of injury outweighs the benefits.

Exercise Progression: One should begin with a weight that can be performed at least 8 times. When 12 repetitions can be completed, the resistance should be increased by 5 percent of the present weight. It is not advisable to increase resistance by more than a maximum of 10 percent between successive training sessions.

Exercise Frequency: The muscle-building process requires about forty-eight hours, so weight training should be scheduled on an every-other-day basis. If you prefer to train more frequently, avoid working the same muscle group on consecutive days. For example, you could work your triceps and chest one day, biceps and shoulders another day, and back and legs a third day. This way you could train six consecutive days a week while focusing more intensely on each muscle group.

CARDIO EXERCISE

Overweight and obese adults may find that accumulating thirty minutes of activity in multiple daily sessions of at least ten minutes in duration is preferable to exerting themselves for longer time periods.

After you are used to thirty minutes of continuous aerobic training, introducing aerobic intervals will enhance your workout. This is done by doing the exercise at a comfortable pace and then increasing the intensity for a short period, then reverting back to the less intense level of exercise once again. For example, you could do six minutes of cardio where you are able to talk with ease at that pace, and then increase your pace for two minutes to the intensity level where it is difficult to have a conversation. After you complete the two minutes, revert back to six minutes of cardio on the previous level; and so forth. You can decrease or increase the intervals based upon your fitness level. The goal of these intervals is to both improve aerobic efficiency and improve your ability to utilize fat as fuel at the faster pace, and to add variety to the exercise program. Please consult a health professional before starting a weight training program or cardiovascular exercises, especially if they are rigorous.

THE HOLISTIC APPROACH

Perhaps the most well-known of Rambam's medical works is his *Regimen of Health* (*Regimine Sanitatis*). In the twelfth century, Rambam's medical writings were studied to understand hygiene. Particularly his *Regimen of Health* was used as a textbook in academies and universities. In 1477, only a few years after the invention of the printing press, a Latin edition of the book was published in Florence. It was the first medical book to appear in print there. Many other editions followed.

Rambam was held in high regard by Saladin and his son al-Malik al-Afdal. He became court physician to Saladin's son after the latter ascended to the throne. As Rambam explicitly states in his introduction, *Regimen of Health* was written at the request of Al-Malik Al-Afdal, who complained of constipation, depression, stress and indigestion. The third chapter is of particular importance, as it contains Rambam's concept of a "healthy mind in a healthy body." The Regimen of Health is filled with psychological and nutritional insights, as well as herbal remedies for stress, anxiety, digestion and optimum health.

All ten of Rambam's medical works are replete with herbal remedies. He did not suggest fad-like herbal ingredients as is common today, but nutritional and herbal ingredients that are considered beneficial and that carry no side-effects even according to modern herbal science. Of particular note, Rambam writes about one of his remedies which he prescribed for al-Malik al-Afdal:

> This anti-anxiety formula should be taken regularly, at all times. It will cause sadness and anxiety to disappear. This is a remedy of which no equal can be found in gladdening, strengthening and invigorating the psyche. It should always be found in your possession.

Rambam believed that maintenance of health should be approached with a combination of mental health, herbal formulations, diet and exercise. Each component is necessary as a combined, holistic approach for achieving effective, long-term results. For a more detailed discussion, please see www.lifetransformingdiet.com.

On the following pages, you will find two sample schedules for Phase 3, if you chose the Light meal (as opposed to the HWC meal) option.

SCHEDULE #1 / PHASE 3

A SAMPLE DAY IN PRACTICE

Begin the day with two glasses of water (cold or hot)

Exercise
20–30 minutes of cardio, plus dumbbell exercises

Breakfast – LIGHT MEAL
Cereal with low-fat milk < 250 calories

Snack – SUBSTITUTION METHOD
Low-fat yogurt

Lunch – MIXED MEAL
Chicken wrap
Two glasses of water midafternoon

Snack – SUBSTITUTION METHOD
Cut up strawberries or other berries

Dinner – ONE CF MEAL
Grilled steak, steamed vegetables, glass of dry red wine

Evening Snack – SUBSTITUTION METHOD
Carrots

SCHEDULE #2 / PHASE 3

Begin the day with two glasses of water (cold or hot)

Exercise – SUBSTITUTION METHOD

20–30 minutes of cardio, plus body strengthening exercises

Breakfast – LIGHT MEAL

2 fried eggs and one slice of toast < 250 calories

Snack – SUBSTITUTION METHOD

Low-fat cappuccino or herbal tea

Lunch – MIXED MEAL

Chicken sandwich on whole wheat bread
Two glasses of water midafternoon

Snack – SUBSTITUTION METHOD

Apple and orange

Dinner – ONE CF MEAL

Grilled salmon and side salad (with optional glass of dry red wine)

Evening Snack – SUBSTITUTION METHOD

Low-fat yogurt

CHAPTER 11
GOAL IN SIGHT

What happens if we break one of our principles or give in to a craving? (I call it "having an excursion.") It may happen at a fast food outlet, at a Shabbos meal, during a weekend afternoon snack or at a family celebration. In fact, it could happen anywhere and at any time. Of course, we have all the information we need in order to combat these challenging situations, but sometimes it is hard to access this knowledge when we need it most. So, what *can* we do if we slip up?

Relax, we all give in once in a while! Don't panic; just calmly get back on track – without berating yourself! It is an expected part of the process of accumulating enough subconscious traces to overcome old habits.

This is not just "motivational talk." This is the way the mind works. The excerpt from *Cheshbon HaNefesh* that we quoted in Chapter 2 bears repeating:

> The sheer strength of "willpower" is inconsequential when compared to an intense desire…if there is a sudden confrontation between these two forces, willpower will be overcome easily.
>
> Nevertheless, due to the kindness of our Creator, the small impressions of willpower are not eliminated completely. Instead, they constantly leave traces which, over time, accumulate so that eventually the strength of willpower increases enough to overwhelm even the most intense desires through this Divine assistance.[1]

1. See *Cheshbon HaNefesh* 56.

In other words, when we stumble it may seem as if all is lost! However, each time this happens, small impressions of the effort we expended to try to overcome that craving are made on the subconscious mind. Although we are not aware of these impressions, they are there. If we choose to continue trying to overcome that bad craving, eventually all the traces of willpower accumulate into a force which is strong enough to overwhelm the craving. If we stay on track, we will succeed and conquer our old bad habit. But we must be persistent and patient, allowing enough time for the subconscious accumulation of traces.

So what can you do practically?

Having two "lapses" a week is built into the system. This does not mean that you should *plan* on having these excursions. Obviously, you will experience more rapid weight loss and quicker accumulation of new, healthier traces if you make fewer deviations from the Life-Transforming Diet. Nevertheless, if you are keeping to the guidelines the rest of the time, if you happen to make two "excursions" in the same week, it will not rock the boat.

However, if you overdo it a third time in a week, then you need to sit down and have a sincere talk with yourself. It doesn't have to be a loud conversation, especially if someone is within earshot! Seriously, it is *vital* to reaffirm your commitment to *your* goal. You cannot expect health, energy and weight maintenance if you are going to eat without clear guidelines and limits. The third time is considered a *chazakah* (precedent) of breaking your desired regimen, and it signals the necessity to get back on track immediately.

It is crucial not to procrastinate. The less accumulation of traces that a new bad habit has set in motion, the quicker you can reinstate your inner, positive equilibrium. Just STOP what you've been doing and get back on track.

Personal Ledgers and Summary Statements are a wonderful way to reaffirm your commitment. Both will be discussed in the next chapter. Personal Ledgers get you back on track and give you a boost, while Summary Statements are especially effective in injecting a feeling of motivation and renewed excitement.

THREE HELPFUL SUGGESTIONS

The biggest problem with taking an excursion from the system is that it will upset your balance of meals. After all, your body cannot tell the difference between a "large snack" and a meal!

1. If your excursion took place at a mealtime – i.e. you ate junk food in a fast food outlet or you ate a full-fat ice cream at an ice cream store for "lunch" – drink water and/or eat only high-water-content foods (fruits and vegetables) until the next meal.

2. If your excursion took place between meals, try to make the next meal a High-Water-Content Meal, even if you already ate one that day. Some excursions are very high in calories and fat. As far as your body is concerned, you have eaten a low-nutritious meal.

These measures are very effective on two fronts:

First, they rectify the "balance of meals" problem. Eating only high-water-content foods until the next meal, or making the next meal a High-Water-Content Meal does not overburden the body. In fact, it injects the body with vital ingredients.

Secondly, these measures serve as an important reminder that there are consequences to your actions. You cannot expect to continue with "business as usual" if you are going to be haphazard in your approach. Most important, get back on track as soon as possible!

231

3. If you overdo it a third time in a week, there is the popular option of getting back onto Phase 2 for three to five days. This will help reinstate your natural controls.

I like to call this measure Turbo Phase. The reason is that Phase 2 is the ultimate mode of the Life-Transforming Diet, according to the guidelines of Rambam. It gives the quickest results and the most cleansing effect. In short, it will get you back on track quickly.

TURBO PHASE (three to five days):

- High-Water-Content Meal once a day

- Fifteen to twenty minutes of cardiovascular exercise plus strengthening exercises, five times a week

- Substitution Method between meals

- Main One CF Meal once a day

- Light One CF Meal once a day

The three suggestions mentioned above are simply good recommendations. They are not requirements.

In a nutshell, until you are down to your goal weight these are the guidelines:

- First lapse is built into the system

- Second lapse is built into the system

- Third lapse requires serious re-contemplation of your goals

GOAL WEIGHT

In *Mishneh Torah*, Rambam writes that if we keep his primary principles of health, we will not become ill and our strength will increase, even if bad foods are eaten.[2] *This will apply when you are down to your correct weight* and your healthy eating practices have become a habit. At that stage, you will be following the guidelines of Phase 3 and will be ready to make responsible exceptions, because your inner controls are strong and in focus. Phase 3 with the potential for making Smart Exceptions is the Maintenance part of the Life-Transforming Diet.

Now, if excursions could remain just that – responsible exceptions – then there would be no need for a method to control them. Unfortunately, we already know that cravings are extremely hard to limit – in quantity and frequency. It is a real challenge to contain an exception!

I will present two methods of making "Smart Exceptions" which will insure that an exception truly remains an exception and not the norm. One method is called High-Cal Exceptions and the other is called Low-Cal Exceptions. High-Cal Exceptions include any food which contains more than 120 calories, and Low-Cal Exceptions include any food which contains 120 calories or less. (Depending on the country in which you live, you will find nutrition data listed in calories, kilojoules, or both. One calorie = 4.184 kilojoules, so 120 calories is about 502 kilojoules.) The Nutrition Label will be explained in Chapter 13. On pages 281 through 283, you will find a list of High-Cal and Low-Cal foods.

In this system, we pay attention to calories when comparing or limiting non-nutritious foods. The only other time we pay attention to calories is when measuring nut or seed toppings or dairy between meals. In these cases, awareness of calorie intake insures that we will not surpass the

2. *Hilchos De'os* 4:14.

definition of a topping or overeat a protein between meals. Otherwise, on the Life-Transforming Diet, the nutritional value of a food always supersedes the calorie consideration.

HIGH-CAL EXCEPTIONS

When you are at goal weight, this method will allow you to make an exception and eat any food or snack *exactly the way you like it*. That's right! It may be a full-fat ice cream at the ice cream store, a regular chocolate chip muffin at a fast food store, Thursday night pizza with french fries, a Shabbos afternoon piece of cake or any dessert at a restaurant. You may have a High-Cal Exception either at a meal or between meals.

The High-Cal Exception is a *planned excursion* once or twice a week – when you are at goal weight. It can be a very powerful method for dealing with constant cravings if you are experiencing them.

There are two ways to overcome some of the strongest cravings: deferral[3] and substitution.[4] By setting a fixed time for your High-Cal Exception, you are implementing both of these psychological mechanisms: You are acknowledging the craving but you are *deferring* it to another time. You also realize that you cannot continue to constantly eat unhealthy fattening foods, as it interferes with your overriding goal of health and weight management. So, faced with a sudden strong craving during the week, you can overcome it by *substituting* this immediate desire with your stronger desire for the weekly or biweekly High-Cal Exception. By keeping to set

---

3. See *Sifsei Chaim, Middos v'Avodas Hashem*, Anger, p. 221, who quotes Rav Eliyahu Dessler regarding deferring an emotion such as anger instead of giving in to it immediately.
4. See *Divrei Yehoshua* 2:2, who writes about overriding one desire by exchanging it for another.

times for these controlled excursions, you will succeed in eating the foods you want without jeopardizing your success. Your desire to look and feel your best will act as a strong incentive – and ultimately the reward – for setting aside any daily cravings.

It is much better to have your High-Cal Exception out of the house. If you must bring it home, try to bring into the house only the amount for that exception. Otherwise, you will find yourself overdoing it, which defeats the whole purpose.

What happens if you make a High-Cal Exception a third time in a week? A third deviation requires serious re-contemplation of your goals. A third time can mean the start of a new habit, so nip it in the bud. Get back on track immediately. Many people find that going on Turbo Phase for three to five days is very effective and motivating.

The High-Cal Exceptions method is for someone who prefers to eat what he or she wants, even if it means only once or twice a week. However, some people may prefer to give in to smaller cravings on a more frequent basis.

LOW-CAL EXCEPTIONS

The four between-meal preferences of the Substitution Method are carefully designed not to ruin the balance of our meals. These options are also based on removing our unhealthy cravings. For these reasons, until you are at goal weight, these are the *only* choices between meals. So while you could eat certain low-calorie desserts in Phase 3, these were not snack options between meals. Similarly, while you could eat a nut topping with a fruit meal, eating nuts between meals was not an option. However, when you are at goal weight, there is a way to eat other foods *between meals* without ruining the balance of meals. These are called Low-Cal Exceptions.

In order to qualify as a Low-Cal Exception, the food should be less than or equal to 120 calories. Sometimes a less nutritious snack between meals, such as an ice pop or a sugar-free ice cream bar, is what you really want. If you are simply not in the mood for the regular Substitution Method or a nutritious Low-Cal Exception – when you are at goal weight – then a 25 to 90 calorie fat-free ice cream or ice pop is certainly a much better option than a 300-plus calorie regular full-fat ice cream bar!

The same applies to other snacks such as a fat-free muffin, a small bag of baked chips or light beer. Obviously, these are neither the most nutritious nor the best food choices, but within the guidelines of Low-Cal Exceptions they offer the possibility of having a responsible Smart Exception.

It is amazing how many low-calorie snack items are available on the market. There are snacks which have less or no added unhealthy and artificial ingredients such as partially hydrogenated oils, colors, flavors, preservatives or sweeteners. Check a product's nutrition label and do some homework so you can make informed choices!

You can choose to have the whole 120 calories at one time, or you may want to split it up. For example, you could eat about 90 calories' worth of nuts and still have room for a nonfat, sugar-free Tofutti pop (30 calories) between meals. But you should not make more than 120 calories' worth of exceptions in one day. (Of course, it is preferable to make exceptions less frequently.)

Remember: it is always best to implement the Substitution Method between meals. Drink, eat vegetables *or* fruit *or* nonfat dairy products, as explained. If you do make an Exception between meals, do not eat the fruit or nonfat dairy options of the Substitution Method before the next meal. Each one of these options between meals is exclusive. However, drinking water and eating vegetables is always allowed.

The key is not to become obsessive about calories. All it takes is a few seconds to determine whether a food can be in the category of a Low-Cal Exception. Is it 120 calories or less? This only needs to be done once with each particular food so that you will know whether it is a Low-Cal Exception.

Now let me remind you that when it comes to Low-Cal Exceptions, *quantity* is of utmost importance. The challenge of a Low-Cal Exception is to control the amount you eat. This goes back to Rambam and his primary principle of food quantity as opposed to food quality.

What can you do if you overdo the 120 calorie mark? You should treat it the same way as you would treat an excursion while losing weight. The first two times a week are built into the system, and the third time requires serious re-contemplation of your goals. Since Low-Cal Exceptions are more frequent than High-Cal Exceptions, it is especially important that you get back on track immediately.

Exceptions are always a challenge. It can take some time before you successfully implement Low-Cal Exceptions or High-Cal Exceptions as a normal part of your healthy regime. After all, every time a person gives in to an unhealthy craving, it can build a stronger inner "unhealthy craving muscle." For some people, it may become very hard to limit Exceptions, and making any type will have to be kept to the absolute minimum. No one is the same, and you will have to see what works best for you. Be patient with yourself.

The key is this: Know that the possibility exists for Smart Exceptions and implement them responsibly. It is important to realize that ultimately no food is out of reach. You have the inner tools and knowledge to handle any eating situation. But long-term success lies in creating and maintaining positive eating habits.

EATING OUT

We have already seen that making the right choices at restaurants is certainly much easier on the Life-Transforming Diet. Here's a brief review of the tools we acquired in the first three Phases:

- If you are having a Main One CF Meal, you can order your favorite steak, grilled chicken, grilled fish or any other main protein dish. Have grilled vegetables or a salad to go with it. Order vegetable soup if you want a starter. (Ask the waiter if they have a plain vegetable soup that is not loaded with oil, butter or artificial ingredients.) If you enjoy wine, drink a small glass of unsweetened wine with the main course.

- A large salad topped with a protein topping, an omelet, a grilled vegetable wrap, pasta (preferably whole wheat) with a tomato-based sauce or a baked potato with olive oil are all popular Light One CF Meal restaurant choices.

- If you would like to have a Mixed Meal, you could choose a baked potato with sour cream, a meat or chicken sandwich, or a main protein course with any starch side dish. Remember, only take seconds of salad.

In the fast food arena, chicken or fish is usually the safest. Salads with a protein topping are also very popular. Always make sure that the dressing is fat-free or low-fat (most regular dressings are very high in fat and calories). Red meat options may not be the best quality. Remember, no fried food.

What about fast food pizza or hamburgers (not homemade)? I feel that these meals should be counted as High-Cal Exceptions. After all, they are low-nutritious meals. Here are some suggestions to limit the damage: When you eat fast food Mixed Meals, the key is to order *moderate* portions with a salad side order (only seconds of salad). For example, try to order one slice (or one and a half slices) of pizza, and a salad or vegetable side order. Order a medium size hamburger (regular bun with ketchup and/or mustard) and a salad or vegetable side order. No high-fat dressings.

GAINING WEIGHT

Both the High-Cal and Low-Cal Exceptions offer effective solutions for making "excursions." Some people may want to mix and match between the two methods. For example, you may want to eat one High-Cal Exception a week and have a Low-Cal Exception every second day. I do not recommend having the maximum of both types of Exceptions every week. Everyone is unique and you will have to see how your body and weight react.

What happens if these measures get out of hand too often? In general, what can you do if you start to gain weight or feel that your health is being compromised?

Remember that every person's weight fluctuates a bit within his or her normal range. But when your trousers or dresses start to feel tight, it's time to nip it in the bud! The worst thing that you can do is to get your clothes adjusted to a bigger size. That would set a self-defeating cycle in motion, and without question further weight gain would follow.

Practically speaking, it is best to get onto Turbo Phase and you will lose the excess weight quickly. At the same time, you will cleanse your body and reinstate that feeling of health and energy. Some people like to revert back to the main guidelines of Phase 2 for one to two weeks. This should be taken as an opportunity to get back to goal weight and return to the new, healthy you.

If going onto Turbo Phase is not effective, try the following steps: Continue the diet at the stage of your particular Phase, but start keeping your

Personal Ledger from the beginning of Phase 1. This can be done by starting the Personal Ledgers from Phase 1, Week 1. For example, if you were up to Phase 2, try to continue with the practical guidelines of your particular week in Phase 2, but start from the beginning of the Personal Ledgers, Phase 1, Week 1. This way, you can pay attention to the build-up of each principle, starting with the HWC Meal and its Summary Statements (see next chapter). In other words, you are trying your best not to backtrack on a practical basis, but you are rebuilding subconsciously from the foundation up. Perhaps your new habits were not firmly established, and all you need is to build a stronger foundation.

If this does not work, you may have to return to the beginning of your particular Phase. If that is still not enough, you may have to start from the beginning of the program, i.e. Phase 1, Week 1. I have seen some people who went back to the beginning of the program two or three times before reaching their goal weight. This was necessary in order to break firmly entrenched habits and set those new positive subconscious accumulations in place.

HEALTH ISSUES

After reaching goal weight, some people choose to start zoning in to certain health issues which are not weight issues.

A good example is artificial sweeteners. Many health professionals believe with absolute confidence that these products are an excellent substitute for refined sugar. However, many people believe that artificial sweeteners should be eliminated or at least limited. If you belong to the latter group, this is the time to start making a change.

(As a side issue, it is certainly not necessary to use artificial sweetener in your coffee or tea because of weight reasons. One teaspoon of sugar or honey is only about 10 to 22 calories.)

A very similar controversy exists regarding caffeine. There are those who believe that within reason, caffeine does not pose a health risk. But if you disagree, this is the time to start making a change.

Some like to go cold turkey off of an unhealthy or addictive product. Others like to move at a slower pace, beginning by skipping days between ingesting them or cutting down on the quantity consumed. Perhaps you will want to substitute an unhealthy product with a "better" version of that product.

For example, decaffeinated products are much better than caffeinated products from an addictive standpoint. So you may want to switch to caffeine-free carbonated drinks for a while. You can then move on to carbonated water with added natural flavor (no calories), then to plain carbonated water, until ultimately you may choose to drink plain water – an unadulterated gift from Hashem which the body needs and enjoys.

CONCLUSION

Once you are down to your goal weight: KNOW YOURSELF! You are allowed High-Cal Exceptions once or twice a week, or a Low-Cal Exception once a day. You may want to alternate between Exceptions weekly, or mix and match in the same week. The key is not to allow the subconscious traces of bad eating habits to accumulate and outweigh your positive eating habits. Certainly, do not allow your exceptions to result in significant weight gain or the need for larger size clothing.

To say that you can never have non-nutritious snacks is unrealistic and a real set-up for failure – especially after having followed the diet so successfully up to this stage. Just knowing that it is not forbidden to indulge occasionally may even eliminate the need to eat unhealthy snacks in the first place. Nevertheless, experiencing a perception change is still the ultimate level of the Life-Transforming Diet. This takes place when you succeed in moving non-nutritious foods out of the realm of your choices, as we will discuss in the next chapter. This is very advanced, and some people may not *want* to reach this level. The High-Cal and Low-Cal Exceptions offer a very effective way for setting healthy boundaries for unhealthy practices.

Once you are down to your correct weight, you will be able to customize your personal eating plan. Of course, no one is the same and we all have different preferences and challenges. For example, some people may choose to make more exceptions and others may choose to be more liberal over the weekends. There are no set rules. However, it is crucial not to fool yourself. You can tell if you are gaining weight or feeling your clothes getting tighter. You can feel the difference between that healthy vibrant feeling when you eat the right foods compared to the heartburn or nauseous feeling, even if you don't gain weight, when you eat the wrong types of foods or overeat. The key is to implement the principles of Phase 3 and try to stay within their guidelines when applying them to your personal preferences.

Obviously, this will not be the case while you are losing weight or initially accumulating subconscious traces for your new, healthier lifestyle. The closer you stick to the exact principles of the Life-Transforming Diet, the quicker you will see results and the better you will feel. This is not the time to be "original" in applying our principles. If you make too many changes, you are simply deceiving yourself. The time to apply our principles more loosely is *only* when you are down to your correct weight or you are genuinely seeing a whole new perspective of how you eat and react to food.

IN SUMMARY

1. *Before you are down to your goal weight,* these are the guidelines for dealing with "excursions":

- The first two deviations in a week are built into the system
- The third time in a week requires serious re-contemplation of your goals

Helpful suggestions to rectify an excursion:

- If it took place at a mealtime, drink water and/or eat only high-water-content foods (fruits and vegetables) until the next meal.

- If it took place between meals, try to make the next meal a High-Water-Content Meal.

- If you overdo it a third time in a week, go on Turbo Phase for three to five days, which will help reinstate your natural controls.

2. *Once you are at your goal weight,* you may choose to eat the following:

High-Cal Exceptions

A High-Cal Exception is a *planned* weekly or biweekly excursion of any food or snack containing more than 120 calories.

A third High-Cal Exception in a week requires serious re-contemplation of your goals. If this happens, you may want to go on Turbo Phase for three to five days.

Low-Cal Exceptions

A Low-Cal Exception is any food eaten between meals which has

Continued on next page

120 calories or less. You can choose to have the whole 120 calories at one time or you can split it up, but you should not make more than 120 calories' worth of exceptions in one day. It is preferable to make exceptions less frequently. If you make a Low-Cal Exception, you may only have vegetables or water until the next meal.

If you overdo a Low-Cal Exception, try to implement the three helpful suggestions mentioned above.

3. In general, if you gain weight or feel your clothes getting tighter, you may want to revert back to the main guidelines of Phase 2 for one to two weeks.

4. On the opposite side of the spectrum, some people choose to start zoning in to certain non-weight issues when they hit their goal weight. Some people will even experience a transformation in how they relate to non-nutritious foods.

5. In a nutshell:

Know yourself! How do you react to making Exceptions? Does it affect your weight or health? Know that the possibility for Exceptions exists, and implement these measures responsibly. Always keep in front of you your ultimate desire for good health and weight maintenance.

No meal or food is out of reach. You have the inner tools and the knowledge to handle any eating situation. Long-term success lies in creating and maintaining positive eating habits, and a continued awareness of yourself and the food you eat.

INSIGHTS AND SUCCESS STORIES

Ronit from England – everything from A to Z

This is not only a book with Rambam's principles. It is not only a book with an excellent diet program. It is not only a book with an innovative perspective on personal development. In my opinion, this book includes almost everything from A to Z in health, and beyond. It is meant to transform your life!

Penina from South Africa lost 18 pounds – realistic guidelines and the power to choose

I don't feel that I am suffering on the Life-Transforming Diet. The system has made me aware of what goes into my mouth and whether I actually want it. I have followed the guidelines and have developed the power to decide what I eat. I have become more aware of when and why I eat the "wrong" things.

One of the most brilliant aspects of the program is that it is realistic. It does not expect me to be 100 percent perfect. Even if I slip up sometimes, I understand that it doesn't mean I'm a total failure. I just take it as an experience that I don't want to repeat. I am so grateful I was given the chance to implement this life-transforming lifestyle!

Rivka from the United States – final stubborn 10 pounds

I lost most of my excess weight on a few different diets. I was feeling and looking much better. But no matter what I did, I could not lose the final ten pounds. I tried restricting myself and would be successful for a few days...but then I'd cave in and lose control. Of course this meant that I gained back the pounds I suffered so much to lose.

This up-and-down seesaw continued until I came across the Life-Transforming Diet. I found this way of eating very realistic and within a very short time on the diet, I finally lost those last stubborn pounds. People are saying I look ten years younger and I feel it!

CHAPTER 12
SEEING THROUGH THE MAZE

THE CREATIVE FACTOR

Rambam writes:

> It is only through the repetition of *actions* that *behavior characteristics* become a fixed part of your personality.[1] If they are positive actions, you will acquire *the good behavior characteristics which motivated those actions.* The same is true about negative actions.[2]

This logic seems circular! After all, we are saying that through an *external act,* you can acquire *the particular emotion which motivated that action in the first place*! Why would you need to develop a motivation that you had in the first place?

Perhaps this is the reason: Although habit may be an extremely powerful force, it can never initiate a new direction. It just follows our existing inner motivations. The underlying motivation must already exist. Only at that point can habits be formed, strengthening the actions which were inspired by the original motivation and preventing an inspiration from fading.

I think this concept sheds light on the fundamental principle which states that "outer actions awaken inner processes."[3] You will notice that it says

1. See *Shemoneh Perakim,* Chapter 4. See also *Mishneh Torah, Hilchos De'os* 1:7 and 1:2.
2. See *Shemoneh Perakim,* ibid. See also *Mishneh Torah,* ibid., 1:7.
3. *Sefer HaChinuch,* mitzvah 16; *Mesillas Yesharim,* Chapter 7.

"outer actions *awaken* inner processes." It does not say that they *create* inner processes.

So the question is: If habit cannot *commence* without a new motivation, how do we *create the first spark of motivation*? In other words, what inner stage usually precedes our emotions?

THE POWER OF PERCEPTION

How can the Torah expect a person to control his thoughts or control what seem to be natural emotions or desires?

One of the great Torah commentators gives the following solution: "You will not desire something which you perceive to be out of the realm of your choices."[4] In *Moreh Nevuchim*,[5] Rambam mentions the same principle:

> Since it is absolutely forbidden to have relations with [close relatives] – punishable by death or excision (*kares*) – men are safe from *seeking* it and their *thoughts* are turned away from it.

In other words, your perception of something has the power to direct your emotions and even control your thought patterns regarding it.

Let us look at a well-known story which clearly illustrates how a sudden shift in perception can trigger completely new and even opposite emotional reactions:

> At the end of World War II, a great Jewish scholar arrived at one of the concentration camps. He went from survivor to survivor, trying to comfort each one. Most of them expressed their gratitude to

4. Ibn Ezra on *Shemos* 20:14.
5. 3:49.

God for being saved. However, one survivor was very angry. He said, "A religious man in the camp somehow managed to sneak in and keep a prayer book. But he would only lend it to those who gave him their daily portion of bread. So every day, he would take many portions of bread from people who were starving, in exchange for the use of his prayer book. After seeing this despicable behavior, I have no interest in religion."

The Rabbi took the hand of this survivor and said to him in a sincere voice, "I understand that it must be so hard for you, but let me make the following suggestion. Instead of concentrating on the one person who demanded a portion of bread for the use of his prayer book, why don't we focus on the dozens of starving religious people, who were prepared to give up their daily ration of food for the use of a prayer book?"

With tears in his eyes the man replied, "You are right, Rabbi. You are right!"

This powerful story illustrates our point. If we choose to focus on the man who was so heartless and selfish, we will see to what depths a person can sink and we will feel angry and upset. However, if we choose to look at the scores of people who sacrificed so much to perform a mitzvah, we are filled with admiration and inspiration. It is amazing that the same story can elicit such extreme and different emotional reactions; it just depends on our perception and interpretation of the situation.

Picture this "candid camera" scene: You are at a kosher restaurant enjoying a meat meal. A worker comes through carrying a box. Suddenly, a piece of ham falls out of the box. At once you drop your cutlery and spit out the food from your mouth.

While this scene is made up, it captures the power of perception. Your food was exactly the same before and after the piece of ham fell out of the box. The only thing that changed was your perception of it. In an instant, you went from enjoying the food to being disgusted by it.

Yet, often we see that a shift in perception does not result in any real change. We continue to eat unhealthy foods even after reading research which indicates that these foods are detrimental to our health. We hear inspirational talks and commit to change but then the inspiration simply fades a few hours later. In other words, why is *perception* sometimes successful in effecting a change and yet other times ineffective?

SHIFT OR CHANGE

Often there is a big difference between a "shift" in perception and a "change" in perception. When a shift in perception takes place regarding a non-personal situation, such as our World War II or kosher restaurant examples, the shift in perception can become a change in perception instantly. There is no opposite, entrenched habit or motivation with which it has to contend. However, when a shift in perception takes place regarding a personal situation, such as your relationship to food or a personal challenge, then the shift must be cultivated and internalized through a new habit. Otherwise, existing entrenched habits or motivations will prevent a change in perception from materializing. This is why it takes a lot of hard work in the direction of your new habit before a real change can be experienced.

Rambam sums it up in his *Moreh Nevuchim*:

> Sometimes we have a flash of insight making the truth as clear as day. But soon after, our nature and habits obscure the truth and we return to darkness.[6]

6. Introduction to *Moreh Nevuchim*.

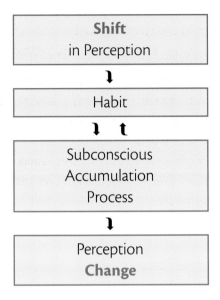

Therefore, real change begins and ends with *perception*. It starts with a *shift* in perception and ultimately ends with a *change* in perception. Yet it is only through habit that we can internalize any new perceptions and motivations. Habit forms the *link* between a shift in perception and a change in perception.[7]

7.   There is another reason why changes in both perception and habit are necessary to make a character change. Let us look at the trait of modesty as an example. *Mesillas Yesharim* (Chapter 23) explains that both perception and habit changes are needed in order to acquire humility. *Sifsei Chaim* explains that outer habitual acts of modesty help instill the character trait of modesty. But what happens if you do not begin by changing your perception of modesty? The outer acts of modesty could even lead to pride, because there is a type of pride which is engendered by displaying false outer acts of modesty. (See *Sifsei Chaim, Middos v'Avodas Hashem*, Modesty 9, p. 150.)

    Clearly, one's shift in perception must be developed through outer habitual acts which reinforce that inner change – and vice versa. One without the other will not be effective. Without a shift in perception, there is no motivation or inspiration to kick-start or direct a new trend. Without habit formation, the motivation or inspiration will soon disappear without ever having developed.

In the Life-Transforming Diet, gaining the knowledge of our principles will cause a *shift* in your perception of physical and emotional health.

Living the Phases creates *outer habits* at the right pace. Simultaneously, *inner habits* are created through the Summary Statements, Personal Ledgers and the re-reading of this book. Both the inner and the outer new habits reinforce your original shift in perception and prevent it from fading. After practicing your new habits for some time, the accumulation of subconscious traces will eventually lead to a *perception change*. At that point, you will *want* to make the right choices, and it is even possible that no inner conflict will be experienced at all.

PSYCHOLOGICAL BLINDNESS

A shift in perception will also give you a picture of where you want to go. It is like a map of the journey to your destination. But a map is somewhat useless unless you are also aware of your current location. I cannot start my journey without joining these two dots together – *where I am and where I want to go.*

In order to determine your current location, you have to make an honest self-accounting: What is my particular situation? This requires a very open mind and a willingness to change. However, bias, self-interest, denial and justification work in our subconscious to reinforce established habits. They make it genuinely hard to actually change no matter how honestly we want to do so. We witness this phenomenon daily. Rambam makes this point:

> Within human nature there is a love and inclination toward one's habits. For example, people of the desert, notwithstanding the difficulties of their lifestyle, dislike the towns and their amenities because they are used to their way of life.

> Similarly, a person has a love for opinions to which he is habituated and he is protective of opinions with which he has been brought up. This prevents a person from recognizing the truth.[8]

> A person seeks opinions which support him in that which his nature inclines. This is true whether it is a result of a natural disposition or an acquired characteristic.[9]

Overweight people assure you, with a straight face, that they "hardly ever overeat or snack between meals." Heavy smokers may proclaim that they "only have a few a day." Alcoholics insist they have a drink only "once in a while." Yet even if we do acknowledge the truth of our habits, the human mind begins to rationalize:

- "It's not so bad that I am overweight because I'm a wonderful, kind person."

- "I don't want to hurt people's feelings, so I end up eating from guilt, frustration, anger or exhaustion."

- "Eating (or smoking) is a tension-release for me. It's the only way I can cope with my stress."

Sound familiar?

This applies to all our bad habits. We often enjoy as well as come to rely on them. We dread the potential short-term stress that might result from any attempt to end them. So without even realizing it, our perceptions and opinions are bent in line with our existing habits.

---

8. See *Moreh Nevuchim* 1:31.
9. See ibid., 2:23.

GETTING REAL

The good news is that if you are reading this book, then you are already on the track of self-awareness. You probably want to make some important changes in your life, and that is why you originally picked up this book. Self-awareness is indeed necessary to gain health and lose weight. If we make an honest self-accounting, we will have a tremendous advantage when it comes to health and weight issues.

Let me put it plainly:

Our bellies do not lie.

Our tight clothing is not an optical illusion.

Any health problems which we may have actually DO exist.

We can try to fool ourselves about weight and health issues, but the evidence is plain to see! (In sharp contrast, when it comes to emotional or ethical issues, it takes a great deal of grueling and honest self-searching to see our inner selves in an objective way.)

PERSONAL LEDGERS

A simple Personal Ledger system is effective in helping you become more aware of what you are eating. Many people honestly believed that they hardly snacked between meals. Others genuinely thought they were following a healthy lifestyle. After filling out Personal Ledgers for just a few weeks, each one came back to me and admitted how unaware they really were of their true eating patterns.

A Personal Ledger achieves the following purposes:

- It records your daily eating, drinking and exercise regimens.

- It is an excellent way to keep track of your progress. It is an indication of whether you are progressing, stagnating or regressing – and at what speed.[10]

- The Notes section enables you to find the source of the delay as well as the obstacles which may be preventing your progress.

- It will motivate you and keep you focused. It works in much the same way as a star chart. Only instead of stickers as a prize, the reward is looking and feeling your best! The Personal Ledger creates a challenge and it tests your resolve. Soon your sense of self respect will outweigh your cravings, whims and moods.

Now, please don't worry! I am not suggesting that you keep a detailed and boring ledger requiring tremendous time, effort and originality. In most cases, all you will need to do is write a number in a box.

How to Set Up a Personal Ledger

The first row tells you which Phase (and Week, if applicable) you are on, as well as your "weekly weight" taken on Sunday *or* Friday Morning (try not to weigh during Phase 1).

The next several rows list each principle, plus provide columns for each day's totals. The final column in each row is the weekly total for each principle.

The last rows are the Notes section.

Here is an example of what a completed Weekly Personal Ledger may look like during Phase 3:

10. See *Cheshbon HaNefesh* 28.

Remember to say your weekly Summary Statement every morning.

Sample Summary Statement:

The "pleasure" of food has become a gateway to obesity and illness.

LIFE-TRANSFORMING DIET — PERSONAL LEDGER

Weekly Weight
Sun/Fri Morning:
158 pounds

PHASE 3

WEEKLY
TOTAL:
6

Principles	Sun	Mon	Tues	Wed	Thurs	Fri	Sat	Total
Continue with: High-Water-Content meal once a day	✓	✓	✓	✓	✓	✓	✓	0
Continue with: 15–20 minutes of cardio and strengthening exercises five times a week	✓	✓	✓	1	✓	✓	✓	1
Continue with: Substitution between breakfast and lunch	✓	✓	✓	✓	1	1	✓	2
NEW PRINCIPLE: **Mixed Meal** OR Main One CF meal	✓	✓	✓	✓	✓	✓	✓	0
Continue with: Substitution between lunch and dinner	✓	✓	✓	✓	1	✓	✓	1
Continue with: *Light* One CF Meal OR *Main* One CF Meal	✓	✓	1	✓	✓	✓	✓	1
Continue with: Substitution after dinner	1	✓	✓	✓	✓	✓	✓	1
How many glasses of water	5	6	6	6	7	5	6	no total

NOTES								
Where	outing		home	home	work	home		
Emotion	craving		craving	tired	tired	angry		
Activity	kids		cooking	bored	stress	kids		
NOTES								
Where					home			
Emotion					tense			
Activity					fight			
NOTES								
Where								
Emotion								
Activity								
MORE NOTES								

Readers are welcome to download or receive Personal Ledgers for every week of the Phases directly through our website, or via email.[11]

THE PERSONAL LEDGER IN PRACTICE

Every night, determine whether you kept to each principle. If you did, put a check in the correct box. If you broke a principle, write a 1 in the box. If you broke it twice that day, you will write a 2, and so on.

At the end of each week, determine the total for each separate principle. The better you keep the principles, the lower your total number will be at the end of the week. Zero represents a perfect score. As time passes and your subconscious accumulation traces get stronger, you will notice that your total numbers will diminish. Once you get used to employing a Personal Ledger, it will take very little of your time. You will never have to spend more than a few minutes each night keeping track of and gaining insight into your progress!

Notes Section

You will notice a Notes section in the Personal Ledger above. If you break a principle during the week, try to determine why it happened and write it down here. This way, you will be able to trace every event back to its source.

Ask yourself the following three simple questions:

- Where was I when I broke the principle?

- What was I feeling when I broke the principle?

11. Internet: www.lifetransformingdiet.com; e-mail: support@lifetransformingdiet.com.

– What was I doing when I broke the principle?

By determining the source of the problem, you might notice that your trigger is external. Certain relationship issues, work stresses or family matters can cause anxieties that "unbalance" us. Other times triggers come from within – a craving or an emotion such as anger or disappointment can overwhelm us. It could also be a combination of external and internal factors. Or you may simply be exhausted or under pressure.

The Notes section especially gives you the opportunity to become more self-aware. By identifying the source of a bad habit, you will be in a better position to avoid, redirect or remove your triggers.

It is best to write no more than three words in the Notes section each time you break a primary principle (see the above example). This forces you to be precise and insures that you will not have to write a long, arduous analysis. You will be amazed at how much these simple notes teach you about yourself.

SUMMARY STATEMENTS

You will notice that at the top of each Personal Ledger, it says: **Remember to say your weekly Summary Statement every morning.**

What is a Summary Statement?

It is a very simple and extremely effective program of contemplation. Contemplation speeds up the Subconscious Accumulation Process.[12] We have already seen how the repetition of outer acts can unleash and transform the inner forces of habit. Contemplation works in the other

12. See *Cheshbon HaNefesh* 22, 25.

direction. It is a very powerful way to effect outer change by the repetition of inner acts. Contemplation forms a direct link between you and your thoughts. It builds a bridge between intellect and emotions.[13] In fact, through this method the subconscious mind can become accessible to the conscious mind.[14] Rambam stresses the importance of Contemplation in his writings.[15] It is also stressed in many other classical works.[16]

I have formulated a method of contemplation, based on principles and methods found in various classical sources.[17] This program is very straightforward and down to earth, and it can take as little as two minutes a day. There are three main steps to this simple but very effective method:

1. At the beginning of the week, choose one or two powerful facts or incentives to create a **Summary Statement.**

For example:

- Overeating is like poison to my body and it is one of the main sources of illness.

- Exercise is a cornerstone in the preservation of health and the prevention of most illnesses.

- Snacking between meals adds up and ruins the correct balance of meals.

- Being overweight is dangerous – physically, emotionally and spiritually.

13. *Ohr Yisrael, Sha'arei Ohr,* Chapter 4.
14. Aryeh Kaplan, *Jewish Meditation* (New York: Schocken Books, 1985), pp. 5–6.
15. See *Regimen of Health,* Chapter 3; *Mishneh Torah, Hilchos Yesodei HaTorah* 2:2.
16. *Hisbonenus* (contemplation) is one of the main themes in the classic ethical work, *Mesillas Yesharim.* See also *Alei Shur,* vol. 2, Gate 2, Chapter 14. See also *Ohr Yisrael, Sha'arei Ohr,* Chapter 4.
17. Mainly a combination of the systems explained by Rabbi Yisrael Salanter in *Ohr Yisrael* and Rabbi Mendel of Satanov in *Cheshbon HaNefesh.*

You can choose a Summary Statement from this book which applies to your weekly principle or which motivates you. Alternatively, making your own personal statements enables you to choose the factors which mean the most to you and have the greatest impact on you. Sample Summary Statements appear on all the Personal Ledgers, which are available for our readers (see footnote 11).

2. For the rest of the week, *every morning*, read the Summary Statement of that week – **aloud**. Then pause for a few moments. Plan how or when you intend to implement the principle or principles of that day.[18]

3. Whenever your mind is free – at home, in the car, on your break – **repeat aloud** your Summary Statement of that week.[19]

The repetition of a concept, mentally and especially verbally, assists in internalizing that concept. It helps engrave the knowledge on your heart.[20] Similarly, the more you read and re-read this book, the more of an impact it will have on you. You will be reminded of the principles, gain new insights each time, feel more motivated and speed up the Subconscious Accumulation Process.

It is also a good idea to **utilize the power of your imagination**. Imagination arouses inner motivations and helps internalize information that was previously confined to the intellect.[21] For example, imagine yourself healthy and at goal weight. "See" how you look; "feel" how confident you are. Notice your exhilaration with your appearance! Imagine all those dreaded illnesses and diseases that you will be avoiding by making the right changes. Feel how much "lighter" you are – physically and emotionally.

18. See *Cheshbon HaNefesh* 22, 35.
19. See *Ohr Yisrael*, Letter 6. See also ibid., *Sha'arei Ohr* 9:3.
20. *Ohr Yisrael, Sha'arei Ohr* 10:7.
21. *Ohr Yisrael, Sha'arei Ohr* 9:2. See also *Mesillas Yesharim*, Chapter 23.

The more **enthusiastic** you are when you study or say your Summary Statement, the more of an impression you will make on your subconscious mind. This in turn will also speed up the **Subconscious Accumulation Process**.[22] Emotions open up the sealed chambers of the heart and allow the waters of understanding to pour in.

In summary, the contemplation program is simple:

1. Every week choose one Summary Statement.

2. Read this Summary Statement aloud every morning.

3. Whenever your mind is free, repeat your Summary Statement.

Utilize the power of your imagination.

Enthusiasm speeds up the Subconscious Accumulation Process.

Very soon, through this program of contemplation, your new insights will start to make a real impact. Remember, no impression goes unnoticed by the subconscious mind. Every inner impression accumulates and will eventually bring about both an inner and an outer transformation.[23]

SHARING YOUR INSIGHTS

During your journey to weight loss and optimum health, it is a good idea to write down your insights, feelings and experiences. (You could use the section at the bottom of the Personal Ledgers called More Notes.) Remember, you can shed light on certain issues in a way that no one else can. There is no one who has your unique perceptions of life. This is why

22. See *Ohr Yisrael*, Letter 30. See also ibid., *Sha'arei Ohr* 9:2.
23. *Ohr Yisrael*, *Sha'arei Ohr* 10:7.

we encourage you to *share your experiences with us*. Use the feedback form below and fax it to us, or you can use the Contact Sheet directly on our website (see footnote 11 for our contact information).

You can remain anonymous. By communicating with us, we will all gain and you will be able to significantly help others who are on the journey you have traveled.

EXPERIENCES, FEELINGS AND INSIGHTS
Name (first or last):
E-mail / Fax:
Country:
Phase (1, 2, 3, goal):
Subject:
Book Chapter:
Comments:

REINFORCING YOUR PROGRESS

Even once you have reached goal weight, you will continue to reinforce your progress. By now, you have made very significant changes. Yet it is important to remember that many of our bad habits and lifestyle patterns were formed over long periods of time. Thus, just as a person who is recovering from an illness will be careful not to cause a relapse, we should also beware of a "relapse" after putting in so much effort. Therefore, the more we can reinforce our new beneficial habits, the more confident and less vulnerable we will be.

Continuing to keep track of your progress using a Personal Ledger is very effective. It is obvious why it plays such an important role during your progression through the different Phases, but once you are at goal weight your Personal Ledger can be just as important. This is because it is easy to lose track of your actual eating habits when you reach your goal – especially if you are making Exceptions. Success has a way of blinding people. Personal Ledgers insure that your eyes stay open.

INSIGHTS AND SUCCESS STORIES

Sandy from England – Personal Ledgers

I am an avid reader of dieting books. I myself never lost weight permanently – until the Life-Transforming Diet. The Personal Ledgers are what help me be aware of what I am really eating every day. At first I thought, "Give me a break. Who has the patience or time? I know exactly what I eat."

How wrong I was! After filling out my Personal Ledger for a few weeks, I couldn't believe what I was actually eating. I could also see what was triggering my eating and bingeing. Soon I wasn't even reaching for the wrong things because I would have to write it down. It really helped me!

I have also greatly benefited from the Summary Statements. They have helped me become aware of and change my unhelpful perceptions.

Leanne from the United States lost 40 pounds – practical advice helps maintain weight loss

I like the practical advice that the Life-Transforming Diet provides. I think that the test of a diet is really how it holds up under pressure. I regularly use the sections that teach me strategies for dealing with temptations that come my way. This has enabled me to prepare mentally for challenges to my eating habits. I also use verbal affirmations a lot! My commitment to a healthy lifestyle has been strengthened and now I have the tools to maintain what I have achieved. Thank You.

CHAPTER 13
NUTRITION: MODERN
AND ANCIENT

SECONDARY PRINCIPLE

By now, it is clear that the Life-Transforming Diet is not about what foods you can and cannot eat. Our program cultivates a life-altering perception which will enable you to eat any nutritious food. In fact, you will eventually be able to even indulge some "responsible cravings." This means that no food will be off limits – if that is what you want. This is because Food Quality is a secondary principle in the Life-Transforming Diet.

The primary principles in our system are Food Quantity (at the meals, between meals and number of meals) and Exercise. Rambam teaches us that if we keep these two primary principles, we are assured of optimum health, weight loss and weight maintenance, even if bad quality foods are eaten.[1] Nevertheless, he still considers Food Quality to be an important principle in a health regimen. As he writes:

Part of the regimen of health is to strive for food quality.[2]

One should choose foods that are digested well and are beneficial for the rest of the body.[3]

1. *Mishneh Torah, Hilchos De'os* 4:14.
2. See *Regimen of Health* 1:6.
3. *Medical Aphorisms* 20:1.

Most people agree that in general, Quality is of utmost importance. Anyone who has a choice between two products that are about the same price will certainly choose the higher quality item. And convinced of a product's superior quality, they will probably spend more money on that item. After all, better quality means better durability and better service.

When it comes to food choices, however, then suddenly – for some unknown reason – the criterion of "better quality" is dispensed with! In fact, some people erroneously think that "dietetic food" means "healthy and nutritious food." This is crazy considering that food is actually put into our mouth and swallowed – affecting every part of the body and mind!

It also amazes me how intelligent people adopt the most outlandishly stringent conditions and illogical restrictions in order to lose weight. Food quality takes a back seat as diets prescribe low-quality foods and even eliminate certain food groups altogether! Now let me remind you that these diets are not suggesting occasional preferences and exclusions. These are long-term preferred food choices and forbidden food groups, based on their principles. Can anyone expect to achieve permanent positive results this way?

The key is to eat a balanced diet – including proteins, carbohydrates and fats. In addition, we should never lose sight of the real purpose of food, which is to nourish and maintain the body. Therefore, beware: Whatever we put into our mouths does not simply vanish. Every part of our body is affected by what we eat. Energy levels, health, weight and even our emotional stability is determined by what we ingest.

REFINED AND UNREFINED CARBOHYDRATES

Carbohydrates are found in foods such as grains, fruit, vegetables, milk, sugars and honey. They are either simple or complex, depending on their chemical structure. Simple carbohydrates have one (single) or two (double) sugars, while complex carbohydrates have three or more. All carbohydrates are broken down and converted into a blood sugar called glucose, and contain four calories per gram.

More important than whether a carbohydrate is simple or complex is whether it is unrefined or refined. In a nutshell, unrefined foods contain vitamins, minerals and fiber. These include fruits, vegetables and whole-grain products. Refined foods lack vitamins, minerals, and fiber. They are often called "empty calories." These include sugary snacks – candy, chocolate and soft drinks, and refined grain products such as chips, white bread, white rice and regular pasta.

What makes the sugar found in candy, chocolate, canned fruits, soft drinks and pastries so unhealthy and fattening? After all, sugar comes from a natural source – sugar cane! The answer is that table sugar is processed and refined to death. During this process almost all the vitamins, nutrients and fiber are removed. What remains are low-quality calories that can only be stored as fat or, at best, provide a spurt of energy. After the sugar is shredded, gassed, heated, spun, sprayed, boiled, dissolved, colored and crystallized, it is easy to understand why natural sugar cane has so little in common with table sugar.

Often, those wanting to lose weight make fat-free products – such as nonfat ice cream – an integral part of their diet. Then they wonder why it takes them so long to lose weight. These "diet" foods may be fat-free, but they're packed with refined sugar! While ingesting less saturated fat is certainly good, nevertheless, the sugars are eventually transformed into fat. So even if you have good intentions, you are merely buying time: fat-free now, but full-fat later![4]

4.   This is where calories count, as I will explain below.

In contrast, the natural sugar found in fruits and some vegetables is unadulterated, and its conversion to glucose is slower.[5] This means that less insulin is produced, which translates into less stored fat. Moreover, most complex carbohydrates are packed with vitamins and nutrients. So first the body utilizes their beneficial ingredients, and only what remains is used for energy or stored as fat.

Like processed sugar, white flour products are highly refined and are taken out of their natural biological context. As a result, they have a very similar damaging and fattening effect on the person eating them. In contrast, whole wheat products contain vitamins, minerals and nutrients. Furthermore, bran, the hard outer layer of grains, is an integral part of whole wheat and grains. Bran is rich in insoluble fiber. When bran is removed from grains, the latter lose much of their nutritional value.

From what Rambam wrote over eight hundred years ago, it is clear that one should eat only unrefined breads:

> Flour that has been sifted so well that no bran remains, or bread that has been kneaded in oil, are bad foods and should not be eaten in quantity.[6]

> Bread should be made from course flour (i.e. not refined flour); that is to say, the husk should not be removed and the bran should not be removed by sifting.[7]

5. Vegetables are a great source of insoluble fiber. Another less known source of insoluble fiber is the skin of many fruits, whereas the inside pulp is a source of soluble fiber. Among its many health benefits, fiber helps stabilize blood sugar levels.
6. *Mishneh Torah, Hilchos De'os* 4:10.
7. *Regimen of Health* 1:6; *Moses Maimonides' Two Treatises on the Regimen of Health*, trans. E. Faris, H.E. Hoff, et al. (Philadelphia: American Philosophical Society, 1964).

Even someone who exercises regularly will become obese if they constantly eat highly refined foods.[8]

THE TRUTH ABOUT FATS

Various foods commonly thought to be unhealthy are actually very beneficial for your body. And some "healthy" foods are actually extremely unhealthy!

Good fats are unsaturated fats that include monounsaturated fats such as olive, canola, and peanut oil, as well as oils found in certain nuts. Polyunsaturated fats are also good fats. They include essential fatty acids called Omega-3 and Omega-6. Omega-3 fats are obtained in fish, flax seeds, and pumpkin seeds. They are also found in smaller amounts in certain fruits and vegetables. Omega-6 fats are obtained from safflower, sunflower and soybean oil.

Bad fats are saturated fats found in *full-fat* milk, cheese, butter, fatty meats and processed meats. Palm oil, palm kernel oil and coconut oil are also considered saturated fats.

The difference between saturated and unsaturated fats is the chemical bonds between the carbon atoms in the fat molecules. Most important, this means that these fats are metabolized differently by the body.

Unsaturated fats can be used positively by our bodies. Among their many beneficial uses, they are utilized by the brain, hormones and nerves. They stimulate our metabolism, strengthen our immune system and help lower bad cholesterol levels, and they can even encourage weight loss. After

---

8. See *Medical Aphorisms* 20:62.

the body metabolizes unsaturated fats, it uses what remains for energy or stores it as fat.

In contrast, excessive consumption of saturated fats leads to weight gain, a rise in bad cholesterol levels, blood clot formation and other health problems.

What about cholesterol?

More than half of American adults have blood cholesterol levels that are too high. This is not surprising, because being overweight contributes significantly to a rise in blood cholesterol levels. While cholesterol is essential for the health of the body, high levels of cholesterol help to form plaque, which builds up and can eventually block the inner walls of arteries that lead to the heart. This increases the risk of heart attack, stroke, kidney failure, blindness and other health problems.

There are three types of cholesterol:

- Low-density lipoprotein (LDL) is bad cholesterol that clogs the arteries

- Very-low density lipoprotein (VLDL), composed mostly of cholesterol with little protein, is bad cholesterol.

- High-density lipoprotein (HDL) is good cholesterol which clears LDL cholesterol from the arteries.

Many professionals believe that the ratio of total cholesterol to HDL ("good") cholesterol is even more important than total cholesterol itself. The LDL-HDL ratio is an even more precise ratio, because total cholesterol is the sum of LDL, VLDL and HDL cholesterol.

It is not unusual to find heart attack victims with relatively low total cholesterol levels, but with a high ratio of LDL-HDL cholesterol.

What part of our diet is the biggest cause of high blood cholesterol levels? One would think that excessive consumption of "dietary cholesterol" is the culprit, but the truth is that dietary fats have a far greater influence on blood cholesterol levels than dietary cholesterol itself. Saturated fats are the main cause.[9] In sharp contrast, unsaturated fats can actually lower bad cholesterol and maintain the good cholesterol in the bloodstream. In this respect, whole-milk dairy products could be worse for bad cholesterol levels than eggs. Though notorious for higher levels of cholesterol, eggs are much lower in fat and saturated fat than whole milk!

For all these reasons, it is crucial to stick to lean meats, chicken, fish and low-fat or fat-free dairy products, and to avoid deep-fried foods. Besides the many health and weight benefits, eating this way will prevent potential health problems.

Trans-fat is the final dietary culprit when it comes to heart attacks and strokes. Trans-fats raise LDL levels and lower HDL levels. In fact, studies at Harvard University's School of Public Health suggest that trans-fats may contribute more to hardening of the arteries than even saturated fat.[10]

What are trans-fats? Trans-fats (also called trans-fatty acids) are fats formed when liquid vegetable oils go through a chemical process called hydrogenation, in which hydrogen is added to make the oils more solid. Hydrogenated vegetable fats are used by food manufacturers because they allow longer shelf-life and give food desirable taste, shape and texture. This process turns even healthy fats into trans-fats, which can no longer be utilized positively by the body. Trans-fat can only cause obesity and illness. The majority of trans-fats can be found in shortenings, stick (or hard) margarine, cookies, crackers, snack foods, fried foods (including fried fast

9. By the way, fat content does not necessarily indicate the cholesterol content. For example, liver is low in fat but very high in cholesterol.
10. Celene Bernstein, *Health Seekers*, audio series, Tape 6.

food), doughnuts, pastries, baked goods and other processed foods made with or fried in partially hydrogenated oils.[11]

A new study reports that when healthy polyunsaturated vegetable oils are used to fry foods, the oils produce a toxic compound that has been associated with a variety of illnesses (including cardiovascular disease, Parkinson's and Alzheimer's diseases) and liver problems. These findings, the researchers say, highlight the risk of reheating oils or reusing them, since the amount of the compound, known as HNE, increases with each heating. The compound forms when the very component of unsaturated oils that is considered so healthful – linoleic acid – oxidizes. The study reported that three other toxic compounds related to HNE had also been found in heated soybean oil.

To make matters worse, many fat-soluble vitamins are destroyed when food is fried. Add to that the trans-fat component, if partially hydrogenated oils are used, and the fact that fried foods are very high in calories and fat.

Is it really necessary to fry food when baking, grilling or steaming can taste as good, if not better? Since I changed my way of eating, fried and greasy food nauseate me. I must admit that when I am eating out, the occasional few french fries are still a weak point, but I keep it that way – *occasional!* At home, when the kids want french fries, my wife places potato slices on a non-stick baking pan coated with a light spray of oil. She sprinkles the potatoes with spices and bakes them in the oven. The kids love it!

Remember these guidelines: Butter is better than most margarines because its ingredients and production are completely natural, whereas margarine contains trans-fatty acids (not to mention the added preservatives, colorants and additives). However, butter should be used sparingly because

---

11. Effective January 1, 2006, the Food and Drug Administration (FDA) requires food companies to list trans-fat content separately on the Nutrition Facts panel of all packaged foods.

it is the number-one source of saturated fat. Whipped or light butter is much lower in fat and calories. Avocado can be used as a spread sparingly. Today, you can even buy some margarines with no trans-fat.

Cold-pressed oils should be used instead of partially hydrogenated oils or oils which were heated during the extraction process. When cooking, it is best to use non-stick pans. If you are going to cook with oil, the best options are oil sprays. Oil sprays come in aerosol or spray pump containers, which eliminate the need to use large amounts of oil. Some of the oil spray brands contain only natural ingredients and are very low in fat and calories. Butter or cold-pressed oil which is put onto already *cooked* food is the best option because the heat is not sufficient to transform the fats.

It is also a good idea to pay attention to vegetarian processed foods. Some of them include hydrogenated or partially hydrogenated oils in their ingredients. The same applies to many common snacks, which are high in trans-fats.

Once again, let us look at a few mind-boggling pieces that Rambam wrote over eight hundred years ago. We will see from his writings that he was clearly against a diet that included the over-consumption of saturated fats and fried foods:

> Fat is completely bad.[12]

> Of the different types of meat, one should choose fowl meat which is not fat.[13]

> Every [type of] fatty[14] food should be avoided...the residue that remains from fatty foods cannot be easily eliminated, and instead it cleaves to the organs. To remedy this, the physician must use strong

---

12. See *Regimen of Health* 1:7.
13. *Treatise on Asthma* 3:4.
14. Literally: thick, sticky, or leaves much residue after digestion.

medications over an extended period of time.... This is very difficult for the physician because the fat remains firmly in its place until it causes the destruction of the organ or the entire body. For this reason, overeating a high-fat diet is sinful and poses a great danger to certain people. It is vital that all the arteries and passageways are open and cleared of obstruction, allowing free flow.[15]

One should choose the lean forepart of the meat, which should not be very fat.[16]

None of a person's food should contain excess fat. Even if one of the good meats described above has excess fat, the fat should be removed except for the amount that makes the meat tasty (i.e. during its preparation).[17]

Some examples of other harmful products include fried pastries and pancakes. Flaky pastries are also very bad because they are unleavened, sticky and inadequately baked. If sugar and honey are also added to them and fried, they are a serious cause of disease.[18]

With regard to preparing animal protein, the most beneficial method is roasting and then boiling.[19]

It is well-known that cheese is a fattening, thickening food, and when it is old it is extremely bad.[20]

Cheese is among the foods that should only be eaten periodically and in small quantities.[21]

15. *Treatise on Asthma* 2:1.
16. *Causes of Symptoms* 20.
17. See *Treatise on Asthma* 3:6 (and see also 3:3).
18. Ibid., 3:1.
19. *Medical Aphorisms* 20:21.
20. *Treatise on Asthma* 3:4.
21. *Mishneh Torah, Hilchos De'os* 4:9–10.

> The best type of fresh cheese is that which is made from milk whose fat has been removed.[22]

These excerpts, which are eight centuries old, have to send shivers down your spine! They were written way before the advent of modern technology, and yet they are amazingly "modern" and accurate. (See Appendix c for more excerpts from Rambam on meat.)

A diet that ignores the issue of healthy and unhealthy fats sacrifices your health, your well-being and also your waistline. Let us pay better attention to what we put into our mouths!

PUTTING CALORIES TO GOOD USE

If you have a choice between a healthy food and an unhealthy food with the same or fewer calories, choose the healthier option. Let me explain.

A large apple has about 90 calories. Three lollipops have about 90 calories. So the "calorie counters" would say, "Equal choice? Go for the three lollipops."

Our bodies react very differently to these two types of foods. It does not mean that there are different types of calories. After all, calories are simply the measure of energy stored in a particular food. However, our bodies first utilize the vitamins and nutrients in the apple and only what remains will be used for energy or stored as fat. There is also the beneficial fiber factor, which we have discussed in detail. In contrast, lollipops provide almost no nutritional benefit – they are empty calories – and can only be stored as fat or at best provide a spurt of energy.

---

22. See *Medical Aphorisms* 20:45. See also ibid., 23:107, where the process of making white cheese is explained.

The same applies to fats. A few small fried chicken nuggets may have the same calorie count as a full size piece of grilled salmon. However, the body can use the Omega-3 fats as well as other nutrients in the fish in a positive way, and only what remains will be used for energy or stored as fat. In sharp contrast, your body cannot utilize the saturated fat in a fried chicken nugget for any useful purpose. And so, it only adds to the bulge and diminishes your health!

Therefore, when choosing foods at a meal, nutritional content always takes precedence over calories. Furthermore, our fundamental aim is acquiring positive eating habits. Constantly counting calories is very cumbersome and psychologically inhibiting. The One CF Meal, Mixed Meal and Substitution Method offer natural ways to insure that you are eating the right quantities both at your meals and between meals.

Nevertheless, sometimes it is important to pay attention to calories. For example, when faced with a choice of which less nutritious foods or snacks to eat, we believe that you should compare the number of calories and choose the lowest calorie option. You are better off indulging in a lower calorie non-nutritious food than a high calorie non-nutritious food.

Interestingly, calories are sometimes an effective litmus test when comparing similar foods or the same foods prepared differently. In this case, the lower calorie option is usually the healthier option. For example, note the fat and calorie differences between eating chicken without skin, with skin and fried.

Chicken (3.2 oz.)	Total Fat	Saturated Fat	Calories
Roasted			
Dark meat, skinless, roasted	8.8 g	2.4 g	186
Light meat, skinless, roasted	4.1 g	1.2 g	157
With Skin			
Dark meat with skin, roasted	14.3 g	4 g	230
Light meat with skin, roasted	9.9 g	2.8 g	202
Fried			
Dark meat, skinless, fried	10.6 g	2.8 g	217
Light meat, skinless, fried	5 g	1.4 g	174
Dark meat with skin, fried	16.9 g	4.5 g	271
Light meat with skin, fried	14 g	3.7 g	252

Salad dressings are another example. Be careful not to fall into the trap of thinking that any salad is a healthy non-fattening option. The type of dressing you use *is* a big deal! For example, when ordering a salad, once you add croutons and a full-fat dressing, you may be having a more fattening and unhealthy dish than one of the other choices on the menu that you decided to avoid!

From a weight perspective, a low-fat or nonfat dressing can make a big difference! Do the math; you will be surprised! However, make sure there are no trans-fats or unhealthy ingredients in purchased, reduced-fat salad dressings.

Salad Dressings	Amount	Fat grams	Total Calories
Fat-free	1 Tbsp.	0	5–25
Light	1 Tbsp.	1.5–4	25–45
Regular	1 Tbsp.	5–9	65–90
Vegetable oil	1 Tbsp.	14	120
Fat-free mayonnaise	1 Tbsp.	0	12
Light mayonnaise	1 Tbsp.	5	50
Regular mayonnaise	1 Tbsp.	11	100

THE CALORIE TEST

Do not be fooled by food products with the label "natural," "sugar-free," "cholesterol-free" or "fat-free." Here is an alarming example:

Which do you think has the highest calorie count?

- Sparkling water with natural fruit flavor

- 100 percent pure orange juice with no added sugar (processed)

- Cola

That should be easy. Cola has almost nine teaspoons of refined sugar in every eight-ounce glass. It must be the worst drink by far! Then the orange juice, because water always has less calories than any other beverage.

Wrong!

Sparkling water with natural fruit flavor often has more calories than commercial orange juice (unless it states "No calories"). I have seen some flavored waters with over 250 calories in a small drinking bottle. But an even bigger shocker is that "100 percent pure orange juice – no added sugar" has more calories than regular cola! Eight ounces of orange juice has 110 calories and cola has 90 calories! Even with all those added heaps of refined sugar, regular cola has fewer calories than some "natural" flavored water and "natural" fruit drinks!

As you see from the figures above, drinking processed fruit juice is not a good idea, especially if you want to lose weight. Furthermore, it lacks fiber and is pasteurized. How can we compare this drink to the "real thing" – I mean fresh fruit! (Not Coca Cola!)

What does this simple example teach us? Not that it would be better for us to drink cola (nice try). It teaches us that not only does "natural" not always mean natural, but that it does not always mean that it won't make us fat.

I will never forget when I experienced this first-hand when I ordered a one-cup serving of "fat-free, sugar-free" soft frozen yogurt. I thought I was eating a non-fattening food; after all, both the fat and sugar content were zero. However, later on that day, I decided to check the nutrition facts. There were 110 calories in every half-cup serving! I also ordered a "fat-free, sugar-free" topping. That added about 50 calories. So it turns out that I wolfed down a "fat-free, sugar-free" frozen yogurt which was about 270 calories. Of course this is not outrageous, but it is certainly not "weight-gain-free." In fact, it has almost the same amount of calories as a full-fat regular ice cream bar!

The chart on the next page is another startling example which helps clarify a widespread misunderstanding. Many people erroneously think that all bread makes you fat. Many types of bread *are* very high in calories. For example, a bagel can have 320 to 350 calories. So it is the calories per serving or too many servings which may make you fat, not the bread itself! Now, compare that to a wrap with 90 to 130 calories, two *light* slices of bread with 80 to 100 calories, two regular slices of bread with about 160 calories or a pita with about 150 calories. A bialy has about 190 calories. Melba toast and crisp breads are examples of much lower calorie options, and they also come in whole wheat versions. Look at the side table for a comparison of other types of breads.

Obviously, it is best to stick to the whole wheat versions of these products. Clearly, the right types of bread are, in fact, very nutritious, and are not high-calorie foods. Moreover, there are many bread options whose standard serving size represents a smaller amount of food.

COMPARE THE CALORIES:

1 bagel (4 oz.) = 320–350 calories

1 bialy = 190 calories

1 slice of challah (2 oz.) = 160 calories

1 pita (2 oz.) = 150 calories

1 wrap (2 oz.) = 130 calories

1 English muffin (2 oz.) = 120 calories

1 matzah (1 oz.) = 109 calories

1 roll (1 oz.) = 84 calories

1 large slice of regular bread (1.1 oz.) = 80 calories

1 slice of light bread (0.8 oz.) = 40 calories

1 crisp bread / Ryvita (0.4 oz.) = 37 calories

1 rice cake (0.3 oz.) = 35 calories

1 piece of melba toast (0.2 oz.) = 20 calories

THE NUTRITION LABEL

How do you measure the calorie and fat content of a particular food item?

Look at the nutrition label located on the package. Here is a sample of a Nutrition Facts label.

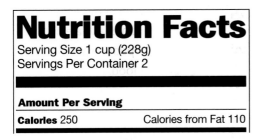

Pay attention to the serving size, particularly to the number of servings contained in the food package. Then ask yourself, "How many servings am I consuming?" (e.g. half a serving, one serving or more). In the sample above, one serving is one cup. If you ate the whole package, you would be eating two cups, because there are two servings per package. That doubles the calories, and in this case you would be consuming 500 calories. (Depending on the country in which you live, you will find nutrition data listed in calories, kilojoules, or both. One calorie = 4.184 kilojoules.)

Limit These Nutrients

In the image on the next page, the nutrients listed first are the ones people generally eat in adequate amounts, or even in excessive amounts. These are the ones to limit. Eating too much fat, saturated fat, trans-fat, cholesterol or sodium may increase your risk of certain chronic diseases such as heart disease, some cancers or high blood pressure.[23]

Total Fat 12g	**18%**
Saturated Fat 3g	**15%**
Trans Fat 3g	
Cholesterol 30mg	**10%**
Sodium 470mg	**20%**

RAMBAM'S LIST

In his *Regimen of Health*, Rambam writes:

> Someone who wants to maintain his health should eat these good foods: wheat bread prepared properly [whole wheat bread], chicken, (low-fat cuts of) meat and eggs.[24]

At this point, I will mention Rambam's list of bad foods as they are found in his *Mishneh Torah*. I chose this list among the many lists found in Rambam's medical writings because it exists in the original and there are no questions regarding the exact translation of the specific foods mentioned here. Furthermore, this list of foods applies to all healthy people, whereas Rambam's specific food recommendations throughout his medical works are often intended for someone suffering from a specific ailment or disease.

Rambam lists[25] three groups of foods that are unhealthy. The first group consists of foods that should never be eaten, the second group includes those foods that should be eaten only periodically and in small quantities

23. For more information, see the first Internet reference for Chapter 13 in Appendix E (page 326).
24. *Regimen of Health* 1:6.
25. *Mishneh Torah*, *Hilchos Deʾos* 4:9–10.

and the third group consists of less harmful foods which should be eaten only in small quantities. In Rambam's words:

> There are some extremely harmful foods that should never be eaten. These include:
>
> ˜ Large fish that are aged and salted
> ˜ Meat or cheese that is aged and salted
> ˜ [Edible] truffles and mushrooms
> ˜ Wine directly from the press
> ˜ Cooked food that has been left until it smells. Any food that has a bad odor or is very bitter is like poison to the body.
>
> There are other foods that are bad, yet not as harmful as the above foods. Therefore, one should eat only a little of these foods and only after intervals of many days. One should not accustom himself to making a meal of them or to eating them as a side-dish with the meal regularly. These include:
>
> ˜ Large fish
> ˜ Cheese
> ˜ Milk more than twenty-four hours after milking[26]
> ˜ The meat of large oxen or large he-goats
> ˜ Beans, lentils, chickpeas[27] (Beans and lentils should not be eaten alone in either the winter or the summer[28])
> ˜ Barley bread or unleavened bread (i.e. matzah)
> ˜ Cabbage, leeks, onions, garlic, mustard and radishes.[29] One should eat them very sparingly and only in the winter, but in the

---

26. In those days they drank fresh milk without preservatives and it spoiled very quickly, especially without refrigeration.
27. Left out of *Kitzur Shulchan Aruch's* list, 32:14.
28. Left out of *Kitzur Shulchan Aruch's* list, 32:14.
29. See also *Regimen of Health* 1:11.

summer one should not eat them at all. (Squash may be eaten in the summer season.)

There are still other foods that are less harmful than the above foods, but they should not be eaten in quantity. These include:

~ Waterfowl and small young pigeons

~ Dates

~ Bread that is roasted[30] or kneaded in oil

~ Flour that has been sifted until no bran remains [white flour]

~ Gravy and (fish) brine[31]

A person who is wise, controls himself, is not drawn after his cravings and does not eat any of the abovementioned foods unless they are needed for medicinal purposes, is certainly heroic.

Remember that Rambam is talking from a nutritional perspective. This does not negate the possibility of recommending some of these foods for medicinal purposes. For instance, Galen writes, "Vegetables such as garlic, onions, cress, leeks and mustard can cure many chronic diseases or at least lessen their severity."[32] Rambam explains several times that a fundamental principle of medicine is that the nutritional effect of some foods is different from their medicinal effect.[33] In fact, he states explicitly in the list above that they are harmful, "unless they are needed as a medicine."

---

30. Left out of *Kitzur Shulchan Aruch's* list, 32:15.
31. Left out of *Kitzur Shulchan Aruch's* list, 32:15.
32. *Galen: Selected Works*, pp. 305–308.
33. See *Regimen of Health* 1:12.

FOOD GROUPS AND OUR PRINCIPLES

It can sometimes be confusing how to categorize foods into the different food groups. The following list will clarify how to define the foods for the Life-Transforming Diet. It will show you how to integrate proteins, starches, non-starchy vegetables, medium-starchy vegetables, fats, fruits, nuts, seeds and legumes into the different meal choices we offer. You will also find a table which illustrates the amounts of a *kezayis* and *kebeitzah* for bread items. An extensive list of Low-Cal Exceptions and how they compare to High-Cal Exceptions will follow.

High-Water-Content (HWC) Meals

VEGETABLES
Non-starchy

alfalfa sprouts, artichokes, arugula, asparagus, bamboo shoots, bean sprouts, bok choy, broccoli, brussels sprouts, cabbage, cauliflower, celery, collards, cucumbers, eggplant, endive, escarole, green beans, kale, kohlrabi, leeks, lettuce, marrows, mesclun, mushrooms, mustard greens, okra, olives, onions, shallots, scallions, parsley, parsnips, peppers (all varieties), rutabaga, spinach, sprouts, summer squash, succotash, tomatoes, turnips, vegetable juice, water chestnuts, watercress, zucchini

Medium-starchy

beets, carrots, peas (fresh), pumpkin, butternut squash, winter squash

SEED TOPPINGS
for vegetables only
(1.5–2 Tbsp. / 0.5–0.6 oz.)

alfalfa, caraway, lotus, poppy, flax, pumpkin, sesame, sunflower, safflower, watermelon

FRUIT

apples, apricots, bananas, blackberries, blueberries, cherries, cranberries, figs, grapefruit, grapes, kiwi, mangoes, melon (cantaloupe, honeydew, watermelon), nectarines, olives, oranges, papayas, peaches, pears, pineapple, plums, prunes, raisins, raspberries, strawberries, tangelos, tangerines

NUT TOPPINGS
for fruit only
(1.5–2 Tbsp. / 0.5–0.6 oz.)

acorns, almonds, brazil nuts, cashews, chestnuts, hazelnuts, macadamia, pecans, pine nuts, pistachios, walnuts

Main Meals[34]

PROTEINS	STARCHES
Meat (beef, lamb, veal), **Poultry** (chicken, duck, goose, turkey), **Eggs**, **Fish** (anchovies, cod, flounder, haddock, halibut, herring, mackerel, pollock, sardines, salmon, sea bass, snapper, trout, and tuna), **Dairy products** (milk, cheddar, mozzarella, Swiss, Parmesan and ricotta cheese, soft cheeses, cottage cheese, yogurt), **Legumes**[35] (peanuts, soybeans, tempeh, tofu, veggie burgers)	**Corn, Potatoes, Sweet potatoes, Beans** (black, kidney, navy, lima, pinto and white), **Chickpeas, Lentils, Green peas, Split peas, Whole grains** (amaranth, brown rice, buckwheat, bulgur, millet, oatmeal, quinoa, sorghum, triticale, whole wheat cereal flakes, muesli, whole grain barley, whole grain cornmeal, whole rye, whole wheat bread, whole wheat crackers, whole wheat pasta, whole wheat sandwich buns and rolls, whole wheat tortillas and wild rice), **Refined grains**[36] (cornbread,* corn tortillas,* corn flakes, couscous,* crackers, flour tortillas,* grits, noodles,* spaghetti,* macaroni,* pitas,* pretzels, white bread, white sandwich buns and rolls, white rice)

35. Legumes and beans are protein and starch combination foods. If they are higher in protein content relative to carbohydrate content, they belong to the protein food group. If they are lower in protein content relative to carbohydrate content they belong to the starch food group.

36. Most of these products, indicated by a *, are made from refined grains. Some are made from whole grains. Check the ingredient list for the words "whole grain" or "whole wheat" to decide if they are made from a whole grain. Some foods are made from a mixture of whole and refined grains.

34. For more information about the "Food Pyramid," see the second Internet reference for Chapter 13 on page 326.

Main Meals (continued)

VEGETABLES
Non-starchy

alfalfa sprouts, artichokes, arugula, asparagus, bamboo shoots, bean sprouts, bok choy, broccoli, brussels sprouts, cabbage, cauliflower, celery, collards, cucumbers, eggplant, endive, escarole, green beans, kale, kohlrabi, leeks, lettuce, marrows, mesclun, mushrooms, mustard greens, okra, olives, onions, shallots, scallions, parsley, parsnips, peppers (all varieties), rutabaga, spinach, sprouts, summer squash, succotash, tomatoes, turnips, vegetable juice, water chestnuts, watercress, zucchini

Medium-starchy

beets, carrots, peas (fresh), pumpkin, butternut squash, winter squash

FATS[37]

Liquid fats: canola oil, corn oil, cottonseed oil, olive oil, safflower oil, soybean oil, sunflower oil

Solid fats are fats that are solid at room temperature: butter, beef fat (tallow, suet), chicken fat, stick margarine, shortening. Coconut oil and palm kernel oil are high in saturated fats and for nutritional purposes should be considered solid fats.

Foods that are mainly oil include mayonnaise, certain salad dressings and margarine.

All fats should be eaten sparingly.

37. Cold-pressed oils can be eaten sparingly with any meal. Butter, margarine (trans-fat free) or avocado can be used as spreads sparingly.

Food Group Criteria

This is the criteria we used above for determining in which food group a particular food belongs:

- **Non-Starchy Vegetable**: Very low in calories, protein and total carbohydrate (less than 2 gm. carb. per 1 oz. serving).

- **Medium-Starchy Vegetable**: Low in calories, protein, total carbohydrate (greater than 2 gm. but less than 3 gm. per 1 oz. serving).

- **Starches**: Higher in calories, lower protein content relative to carbohydrate content, high total carbohydrate (greater than 3 gm., up to 18 gm. per 1 oz. serving).

- **Proteins**: High in protein either by itself or relative to carbohydrate content.

Applying the Food Groups to Our Main Meal Principles

- **HWC Meal**: Eat a vegetable meal with a low-fat dressing and an optional seed topping, OR a fruit meal with an optional nut topping.

- **One CF Meal:**
  - Protein with **non-/medium-starchy vegetables**

  OR

  - Starches with **non-/medium-starchy vegetables**

- **Mixed Meal**: Any combination of foods (except fruit), but only take seconds of salad and vegetables.

KEZAYIS AND KEBEITZAH

This table illustrates the bread amounts of a *kezayis* and *kebeitzah*:[38]

TYPE	KEZAYIS		KEBEITZAH	
Bagel	⅒ of a bagel	13 grams	⅕ of a bagel	26 grams
Rye Bread – small 1 lb. loaf	½ of center slice	10 grams	1 slice	20 grams
Rye Bread – large 2 lb. loaf	¼ of center slice	10 grams	½ slice	20 grams
White bread	⅓ slice	8 grams	⅔ slice	16 grams
Challah roll	⅑ of a roll	5 grams	¼ of a roll	10 grams
Matzah	4/10 of a matzah	15 grams	¾ of a matzah	30 grams
Onion roll	⅒ of a roll	6 grams	⅕ of a roll	12 grtams
Pita bread	¼ of a pita	12 grams	½ of a pita	24 grams
Flat bread	1¾ pieces	19 grams	3½ pieces	38 grams

LOW-CAL AND HIGH-CAL EXCEPTIONS

Below you will see a list of some examples of High-Cal and Low-Cal Exceptions. Foods with 120 calories or less are highlighted in grey. Foods with more than 120 calories are not highlighted. Of course, the list is not conclusive.

38. See Rabbi Yisroel Bodner, *Halachos of K'zayis* (Jerusalem: Feldheim Publishers, 2001), pp. 82–88.

Smart Exception	Amount	Fat grams	Total Calories
Ice Cream			
Ice pops	1	0	20–50
Fruit ice pops	1	0	80
Sorbet	½ cup (4 fl. oz.)	0	90–120
Frozen yogurt	½ cup (4 fl. oz.)	0–3	100–120
Low-fat/nonfat ice cream	½ cup (4 fl. oz.)	0–4	90–120
Regular ice cream	½ cup (4 fl. oz.)	7–18	130–270
Regular ice cream bar	1	10–35	210–375
Cookies and Pastries			
Crackers	1 average	1	20
Small chocolate chip cookies	1	2	35
Fat-free muffins	1	0	80
Muffins	1 (3 oz.)	10	240
Doughnut	1 (2 oz.)	11–14	210–260
Brownie, frosted	1	9	180
Cookie (large)	1 (2.3 oz.)	12–16	280–310
Chocolate			
Small-bite chocolates	1	1.5	25
Low-calorie bar	1	0	120
Average chocolate bar	2 oz.	20	300
Chocolate-covered nuts	1 pack (1.5 oz.)	13	230
Candies and Snacks			
Hard candies	1	0	9–18
Lollipop	1	0	30
Gum	1	0	5–35
Fruit leather	1	0	45
Licorice (twists)	1 piece	0	30

Continued on next page

Smart Exception	Amount	Fat grams	Total Calories
Homemade popcorn (made without oil)	1 oz. (3½ cups)	0–1	100
Marshmallows	6 (regular size)	0	100
Licorice	1 oz.	0	100
Toffee	1 oz. (regular)	9	150
Halvah	1 bar (4 oz.)	50	780
Chips			
Potato chips (fat-free)	1 oz. package	0	70–100
Potato chips (baked)	1 oz. package	1.5–3	110
Potato chips (reduced fat)	1 oz. package	6–8	140–150
Potato chips (regular)	1 oz. package	10–11	150–160
Onion rings	1 oz. package	6	140
Pretzels			
Pretzels (fat-free)	1 oz.	0–1	100–110
Pretzels (hard-baked)	1 oz.	2	110
Pretzels (coated)	1 oz.	6	140
Drinks			
Water (plain), seltzer (plain, calorie-free), diet soda, tea and coffee[39]	unlimited	0	0
Vegetable juice	1 cup (8 fl. oz.)	0	50–60
Wine	4 fl. oz.	0	80–100
Fruit juice	1 cup (8 fl. oz.)	0	110
Soy milk (plain)	1 cup (8 fl. oz.)	0–5	60–120
Cow's milk (plain) – nonfat, 1%, 2%	1 cup (8 fl. oz.)	0–5	90–120
Liquor	1 shot (1 fl. oz.)	0	65–85

Continued on next page

39. Not more than one or two teaspoons of sugar in coffee or tea. More than this counts toward a Low-Cal Exception.

Smart Exception	Amount	Fat grams	Total Calories
Beer (light)	1 can (12 fl. oz.)	0	70–120
Reduced-calorie soda	1 can (12 fl. oz.)	0	85
Iced tea (sweetened)	1 can (12 fl. oz.)	0	90–165
Beer (regular)	1 can (12 fl. oz.)	0	160–200
Regular soda	1 can (12 fl. oz.)	0	150
Flavored milk, milkshake	1 cup (8 fl. oz.)	0–9	120–300
Dairy			
Fat-free cheese	1 slice (1 oz.)	0	50
Low-fat cheese	1 slice (1 oz.)	1.5	50
Light cheese	1 slice (1 oz.)	5	80
Cheese stick, light	1 stick	5	80
Plain yogurt, nonfat	1 cup (8 oz.)	0	80–100
Low-fat yogurt	1 cup (8 oz.)	4	140
Whole-fat yogurt	1 cup (8 oz.)	7	180
Nuts[40] and Seeds			
Pistachios (shelled)	½ oz. (22 nuts)	7	80
Sunflower seeds	½ oz. (⅛ cup)	7	80
Almonds	½ oz. (13 medium)	7.5	85
Pecans	½ oz. (15 large halves)	9	95
Cashews	½ oz. (13 small)	7	80
Walnuts	½ oz. (10 halves)	8	88
Macadamia	½ oz. (7 small)	10	100

40. It is a good idea to choose small nuts and the ones that will allow you to eat as many as you can within your calorie target. This will leave you feeling far more satisfied. Remember: Raw is better than roasted, dry-roasted is better than honey-roasted, honey-roasted is better than oil-roasted and oil-roasted is better than coated nuts.

The above list provides the average nutritional information for these foods. However, there are many different brands, and each one may have a different calorie and fat content. So check the nutrition label to see if a particular food falls within the category of a Low-Cal or a High-Cal Exception. It will take only a few minutes, and it only needs to be done once for each food.

Remember: When it comes to Low-Cal Exceptions, *quantity* is of utmost importance. The challenge of a Low-Cal Exception is to control the amount you eat. This goes back to Rambam's Primary Principle of Food Quantity as opposed to his Secondary Principle of Food Quality.

Beware: Smart Exceptions – both High-Cal and Low-Cal – only become a possibility after you are at goal weight. You are risking the effectiveness of this whole program if you try to make these exceptions before then. After all, one of the main goals of the Phases is to realign your inner controls, and this is impossible if you are making too many exceptions. However, when you are ready, Smart Exceptions can be very effective in insuring that exceptions remain exceptions.

IN SUMMARY

- Try to choose unrefined foods over refined foods
- Try to choose low-fat foods over high-fat foods, which includes no heated fats or trans-fats
- Compare the amount of calories in non-nutritious items
- Low-Cal Exceptions: less than or equal to 120 calories (not more than once a day)
- High Cal Exceptions: any food or meal once or twice a week
- Pay attention to Rambam's bad food list
- Avoidance: Try to keep the house full of nutritious foods

Our aim is to transform our relationship with food in a conscious and subconscious way. This is evident in those who have successfully followed the system. Some who have never been able to get down to normal weight have been literally transformed on this program! Best of all, they have kept the weight off. Truthfully, it is relatively easy to lose some weight on any diet, but the Life-Transforming Diet can help you go all the way and stay there!

INSIGHTS AND SUCCESS STORIES

Chana from the United States lost over 25 pounds – spends hours in the kitchen

I spend many hours a day in the kitchen. I was tired of all the usual diets, because so many of my favorite foods were out of bounds. So I just started to accept that I would probably be overweight for the rest of my life.

When I was introduced to the Life-Transforming Diet, I could not believe that the final Phase would allow me to snack between meals. I also learned practical ways to deal with my old indulgences. I realized that this approach was totally different from all the other diets that I had tried. I decided to give it a chance.

I have lost a lot of weight and I love how I feel and look. I honestly think that the way I view food has been transformed. I can spend many hours a day in the kitchen and feel confident with the way I relate to food. Amazingly, by the time I reached the final Phase, I did not feel a need to constantly snack. In fact, I no longer enjoy artificial, sweet-tasting foods. Yet just knowing that they are not totally forbidden is very liberating.

THE LIFE-TRANSFORMING DIET QUICK REFERENCE

(The word **Add** indicates that you should begin a new principle but also continue with the previous principle/s.)

PHASE 1

Week 1
High-Water-Content Meal once a day

Week 2
Add: 5–10 minutes of cardiovascular exercise five times a week

Week 3
Add: Substitution Method between meals

Week 4
Add: Main One CF Meal for the main meal

Week 5
Add: Light One CF Meal for the remaining meal

PHASE 2

Week 1
Add: Move up to 10–15 minutes of cardiovascular exercises and add basic strengthening exercises, five times a week

Week 2
Reinforce the previous Guidelines

Week 3
Add: Move up to 15–20 minutes of cardiovascular exercises and add more advanced strengthening exercises, five times a week

PHASE 3
Follow until Goal Weight

Add: Mixed Meal once a day – **Take seconds of vegetables only.**
Add: More dessert options (ranging from 0 calories to 90 calories)
  – Option to increase cardiovascular and strengthening exercises

AT GOAL WEIGHT

  – **Low-Cal Exceptions** ≤ 120 Calories, not more than once a day

OR

  – **High-Cal Exceptions** > 120 calories, once or twice a week

IN A NUTSHELL

To sum up our main nutritional principles:

Meals, from Phase 3
~ One meal should always be a High-Water-Content Meal.
~ The main meal could either be a Main One CF Meal or a Mixed Meal.
~ Suggestion: If your largest meal is a Main One CF Meal, you can make the other meal a Mixed Meal. If your largest meal is a Mixed Meal, you should try to make the other meal a Light One CF Meal.

Between meals
~ First preference: Drink (water, seltzer, herbal tea, decaf coffee or diet soda)
~ Second preference: Vegetables
~ Third preference: Fruit
~ Fourth preference: Non/low-fat dairy products (≤ 90 calories)
~ At goal weight: Fifth preference: Low-Cal Exceptions or High-Cal Exceptions

Remember, each one of these options between meals is exclusive and cannot be eaten together. The exception is vegetables, which is always an option between meals.

Dessert options
~ Phases 1 and 2: A small amount of unsweetened applesauce or constipating fruits
~ Phase 3: Low-calorie dessert options, ranging from 0 to 90 calories
~ At goal weight: Low-Cal Exceptions or High-Cal Exceptions, as explained above

DEALING WITH EXCURSIONS AND SMART EXCEPTIONS

* *Before you are down to your goal weight*, these are the guidelines for dealing with "excursions": The first two deviations in a week are built into the system. The third time in a week requires serious re-contemplation of your goals.

Helpful suggestions to rectify an excursion:
~ If it took place at a mealtime, drink water or eat only high-water-content foods (fruits and vegetables) until the next meal.
~ If it took place between meals, try to make the next meal a High-Water-Content Meal.
~ If you overdo it a third time in a week, go on Turbo Phase for three to five days, which will help reinstate your natural controls.

* *Once you are at your goal weight*, you may choose to eat the following:

HIGH-CAL EXCEPTIONS:
A third High-Cal Exception in a week requires serious re-contemplation of your goals. Many people like to go on Turbo Phase for three to five days.

LOW-CAL EXCEPTIONS:
If you overdo a Low-Cal Exception, try to implement the three helpful suggestions mentioned above.

APPENDIX A
BODY MASS INDEX (BMI)

BMI AND YOU

In general, overweight is defined as one to thirty pounds over your healthy weight. Obesity is defined as being thirty pounds or more over your healthy weight. However, for a more precise measure, the Body Mass Index (BMI) was introduced. It is a ratio which measures weight relative to height. It indicates the level of body fat better than any other gauge.

The present definitions of healthy weight, overweight and obesity were established after numerous studies compared the BMIs of millions of people and compared them with the rates of illness and death.

Keep in mind that BMI is only one factor related to risk for disease. For assessing someone's likelihood of developing overweight- or obesity-related diseases, the National Heart, Lung, and Blood Institute guidelines recommend looking at two other predictors:

— The individual's waist circumference (because abdominal fat is a predictor of risk for obesity-related diseases).

— Other risk factors the individual has for diseases and conditions associated with obesity (for example, high blood pressure or physical inactivity).

CALCULATING BMI[1]

BMI is calculated the same way for both adults and children. The calculation is based on the following formulas:

Measurement units	Formula and calculation
Kilograms and meters (or centimeters)	**FORMULA: weight (kg.) ÷ [height (m.)]²** With the metric system, the formula for BMI is weight in kilograms divided by height in meters squared. Since height is commonly measured in centimeters, divide height in centimeters by 100 to obtain height in meters. EXAMPLE: Weight = 68 kg., Height = 165 cm. (1.65 m.) CALCULATION: $68 \div (1.65)^2 = 24.98$
Pounds and inches	**FORMULA: [weight (lb.) ÷ (height [in.])²] × 703** Calculate BMI by dividing weight in pounds by height in inches squared, and then multiplying by a conversion factor of 703. EXAMPLE: Weight = 150 lbs., Height = 5'5" (65") CALCULATION: $[150 \div (65)^2] \times 703 = 24.96$

---

1. For more information regarding BMI, see the first Internet reference for Appendix A on page 326.

BMI CHART

1. Find your *height* in the left column of the BMI Chart.

2. Follow it across to find the weight that is closest to your body weight.

3. Then work your way up to find your *Body Mass Index* (BMI).

BMI	19	20	21	22	23	24	25	26	27	28	29	30	31	32	33	34	35
Height (in feet/ inches)							Weight (in pounds)										
4'10"	91	96	100	105	110	115	119	124	129	134	138	143	148	153	158	162	167
4'11"	94	99	104	109	114	119	124	128	133	138	143	148	153	158	163	168	173
5'0"	97	102	107	112	118	123	128	133	138	143	148	153	158	163	168	174	179
5'1"	100	106	111	116	122	127	132	137	143	148	153	158	164	169	174	180	185
5'2"	104	109	115	120	126	131	136	142	147	153	158	164	169	175	180	186	191
5'3"	107	113	118	124	130	135	141	146	152	158	163	169	175	180	186	191	197
5'4"	110	116	122	128	134	140	145	151	157	163	169	174	180	186	192	197	204
5'5"	114	120	126	132	138	144	150	156	162	168	174	180	186	192	198	204	210
5'6"	118	124	130	136	142	148	155	161	167	173	179	186	192	198	204	210	216
5'7"	121	127	134	140	146	153	159	166	172	178	185	191	198	204	211	217	223
5'8"	125	131	138	144	151	158	164	171	177	184	190	197	203	210	216	223	230
5'9"	128	135	142	149	155	162	169	176	182	189	196	203	209	216	223	230	236
5'10"	132	139	146	153	160	167	174	181	188	195	202	209	216	222	229	236	243
5'11"	136	143	150	157	165	172	179	186	193	200	208	215	222	229	236	243	250
6'0"	140	147	154	162	169	177	184	191	199	206	213	221	228	235	242	250	258
6'1"	144	151	159	166	174	182	189	197	204	212	219	227	235	242	250	257	265
6'2"	148	155	163	171	179	186	194	202	210	218	225	233	241	249	256	264	272
6'3"	152	160	168	176	184	192	200	208	216	224	232	240	248	256	264	272	279
6'4"	156	164	172	180	189	197	205	213	221	230	238	246	254	263	271	279	287

To convert from kilograms to pounds, multiply the kilograms by 2.2.

To convert from meters to inches, divide the meters by 0.0254.

INTERPRETATION OF BMI FOR ADULTS

For adults twenty years and older, BMI is interpreted using standard weight status categories that are the same for all ages and for both men and women. They are shown in the following table:

BMI	WEIGHT STATUS
Below 18.5	Underweight
18.5 to 24.9	Normal
25.0 to 29.9	Overweight
30.0 and above	Obese

For example, here are the weight ranges, the corresponding BMI ranges, and the weight status categories for a sample height.

HEIGHT	WEIGHT RANGE	BMI	WEIGHT STATUS
5'9"	124 lbs. or less	Below 18.5	Underweight
	125 lbs. to 168 lbs.	18.5 to 24.9	Normal
	169 lbs. to 202 lbs.	25.0 to 29.9	Overweight
	203 lbs. or more	30 and above	Obese

BMI FOR CHILDREN

Although the BMI number is calculated the same way for children as for adults, the criteria used to interpret the meaning of the BMI number for children and teens are different from those used for adults. For children and teens, BMI age- and sex-specific percentiles are used for two reasons:

- The amount of body fat changes with age

- The amount of body fat differs between girls and boys

This is how some sample BMI numbers would be interpreted for a ten-year-old boy.

BMI	PERCENTILE IN BMI-FOR-AGE CHART	WEIGHT STATUS
13	Less than 5th percentile	Underweight
18	5th to less than 85th percentile	Normal
21	85th to less then 95th percentile	At risk
23	95th percentile or greater	Overweight

OTHER EXCEPTIONS

BMI is not always an accurate way to determine ideal weight. Here are some exceptions:[2]

- **Body builders:** Because muscle weighs more than fat, people who are unusually muscular may have a high BMI.

- **The elderly:** In the elderly it is often better to have a BMI between 25 and 27, rather than under 25. If you are over sixty-five, for example, a slightly higher BMI may help protect you from osteoporosis.

2. For more information, see the second Internet reference for Appendix A on page 326.

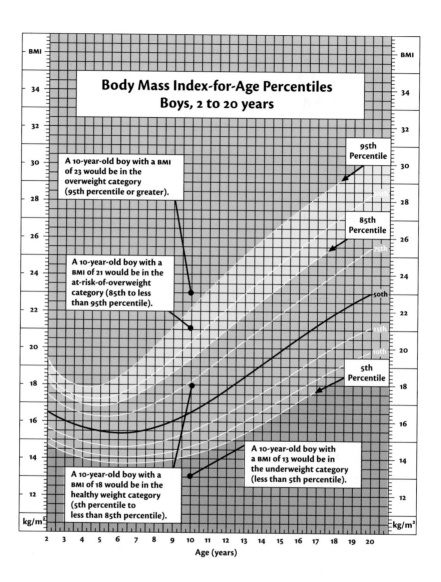

BMI

34

32

30

28

26

24

22

20

18

16

14

12

kg/m²

**Body Mass Index-for-Age Percentiles
Boys, 2 to 20 years**

A 10-year-old boy with a BMI of 23 would be in the overweight category (95th percentile or greater).

A 10-year-old boy with a BMI of 21 would be in the at-risk-of-overweight category (85th to less than 95th percentile).

A 10-year-old boy with a BMI of 18 would be in the healthy weight category (5th percentile to less than 85th percentile).

A 10-year-old boy with a BMI of 13 would be in the underweight category (less than 5th percentile).

95th Percentile

85th Percentile

5th Percentile

90th

75th

50th

25th

10th

BMI

34

32

30

28

26

24

22

20

18

16

14

12

kg/m²

2 3 4 5 6 7 8 9 10 11 12 13 14 15 16 17 18 19 20

Age (years)

304

APPENDIX B
A SHORT BIOGRAPHY
OF RAMBAM

Rambam was a sage and a genius. Any attempt to summarize who and what he was and is, in a few lines, is futile. Rambam was almost "superhuman." Volumes have been written on his life and works, and his greatness is beyond our comprehension. All I offer you is a very brief bird's eye view of this truly great man, with a special emphasis on his medical contribution to society.

Rambam lived in dangerous times and through many persecutions and personal tragedies. Nonetheless, he became a world-renowned expert in the subjects of theology, law, medicine, philosophy, psychology, mathematics, languages and astronomy.

Rambam was a prolific author and wrote many comprehensive sets of books which include every area of thought. Each one of his works was brilliant enough to have assured him a prominent place in the pages of history. To this day, his style of precision, depth, clarity and "simplicity" is unparalleled.

While most of Rambam's works on law, philosophy and ethics are well-known and studied to this day, his many medical writings are not as well-known and are more difficult to access.

Rambam placed great emphasis on the subject of medicine. One of the many examples is found in his *Shemoneh Perakim*:[1]

---

1. Chapter 5.

> Medical knowledge is an extremely important prerequisite for intellectual and personal development, the knowledge of God and the attainment of true success. Its study and practice should be considered among the great duties, and it should not be considered simply as one of the working trades. Medical knowledge directs our conduct and leads to genuine personal development.

Rambam was held in high regard by Saladin and his son al-Malik al-Afdal. Rambam became court physician to Saladin's son after the latter ascended to the throne. It is said that at around the same time, he was invited to be the personal physician to the famous Richard the Lionheart. In his later years he was considered to be the greatest physician of his time. As the world-renowned physician Sir William Osler so aptly said, "Maimonides was the Prince of Physicians."

There was a time in history when Rambam's medical works enjoyed extreme popularity throughout the world. In the twelfth century his medical writings were studied to understand hygiene. During the Middle Ages, his *Regimen of Health* was used as a textbook in academies and universities. In 1477, only a few years after the invention of printing, a Latin edition was published in Florence; it was the first medical book to appear in print there. Many other editions followed.

Ibn Abi Ozeibia (1203–1270), the most famous Arab physician and historian of Cairo, concludes his bibliography of Rambam with a famous poem describing Rambam as a healer of the body and the mind, as apposed to Galen who was only a physician of the body. Abd al-Latif, a famous physician at that time, specifically traveled to Cairo to see Rambam with his own eyes.[2]

---

2.   Rambam, *Hanhagot HaBriut*, trans. S. Munter (Jerusalem: Mosad Harav Kook, 1957), Introduction.

Waldmer Schweiseheimer, a mid-twentieth century historian, said of Rambam's medical writings, "Rambam's medical teachings are not antiquated at all. His writings, in fact, are in some respects astonishingly modern in tone and contents."[3]

To me, Rambam represents the pursuit of absolute truth. He was not afraid to disagree with the greatest minds or agree with his biggest opponents. This approach was extremely controversial and even dangerous in his time, when very little intellectual or religious tolerance existed.

Rambam is often referred to as the "Great Eagle," for he carried his people upon his wings. In his time, the Karaites,[4] as well as the intense belief in secular philosophy and forcible conversion by the sword, threatened to uproot the foundations of our belief. Rambam taught his people how to overcome and channel these trials as a growing experience through his uncompromising Torah perspective. Dealing with the issues of his time, many of which are still very relevant today, Rambam continues to serve as a beacon of light and a "great eagle." To this day, Rambam's name stands for the highest intellectual and spiritual accomplishments. The famous adage, which is engraved on his tombstone, sums up the greatness of the man perfectly:

From Moshe to Moshe there never arose a man like Moshe.

After his death Rambam was mourned throughout the world by all sects of religion. In fact, there was a general three-day mourning period in Egypt.

3. Encyclopedia Britannica, "Moses Rambam."
4. A sect which denied Rabbinical tradition. In Rambam's time they comprised about 30 percent of the Jewish world population. In Egypt, they were a majority.

APPENDIX C
RAMBAM AND MEAT

> The commandment concerning the slaughtering of animals is
> necessary. For the natural food of man consists only of the plants
> deriving from seeds growing in the earth and of the flesh of animals,
> the most excellent kinds of meat being those that are kosher. No
> physician is ignorant of this. Now since the necessity to have good
> food requires that animals be killed, the aim was to kill them in the
> easiest manner.[1]

The excerpts in this appendix have been gathered from many of Rambam's
different works.

CHICKEN

Throughout his medical works, Rambam writes about many different
health benefits that result from eating the different types of fowl:[2]

> Of the different types of meat, one should choose fowl meat which
> is not fatty.[3]

> Fowl is easily digested.[4]

1. *Moreh Nevuchim* 3:48.
2. See *Regimen of Health* 4:16 and *Medical Aphorisms* 20:68 and 20:69.
3. *Treatise on Asthma* 3:4.
4. *Medical Aphorisms* 20:20.

In general, the meat of birds is lighter than the meat of cattle and is more quickly digested.[5]

One should not eat even of the best types of meat unless one becomes bored with chicken.[6]

Of the chicken species, one should not take those that are more than two years old, too young, too lean or those fattened by force-feeding. The manner of their management is as follows: The chickens should be let loose on spacious grounds in which there is no dirt or garbage. The area should be cleaned regularly. They should be fed a quantity that fills their crops.[7]

Someone who wants to maintain his health should eat these beneficial foods:...chicken, pheasant,[8] pigeons and turtledoves.

Choose fowl meat which is not fat...such as francolin,[9] pigeon[10] and partridge.[11]

All waterfowl like geese and duck are harmful foods.[12]

The physicians have mentioned that chicken soup has many healing properties.[13]

Boiled chicken soup stabilizes body constitution and it is an excellent food and medication for treating ailments and diseases.[14]

---

5. *Regimen of Health* 1:7.
6. *Causes of Symptoms* 20; See also *Mishneh Torah, Hilchos De'os* 5:10.
7. *Causes of Symptoms* 20.
8. Some translate partridge.
9. Some translate hazel hen.
10. Some translate turtledove.
11. *Treatise on Asthma* 3:4.
12. Literally: thick and contain many harmful humors; *Treatise on Asthma* 3:4.
13. *Causes of Symptoms* 20.
14. See *Medical Aphorisms* 20:68 and 20:83.

RED MEAT

All meats aren't of the same nature or equally beneficial.[15]

One should avoid all fatty meats like that of cattle, goats and grown sheep. Galen said that the latter meats are worse than the meat of cattle.[16]

Someone who wants to maintain his health should eat these beneficial foods: ...the meat of a kid, a one-year-old lamb.[17]

Kid meat is exceptionally good, more so than the meat of any other animal.[18]

Goats and old cows are bad fatty foods.[19]

One should not eat stall-fed sheep, especially the fat ones.[20]

Lamb is not good nourishment (except for the one-year-old lamb).[21]

Meat that is aged and salted should never be eaten.[22]

The Best Cuts

One should choose the *lean forepart of the meat*, which should not be very fat.[23]

---

15. See *Regimen of Health* 1:7.
16. *Treatise on Asthma* 3:3.
17. See *Regimen of Health* 1:6 and 1:7; See also *Medical Aphorisms* 20:70.
18. *Medical Aphorisms* 20:70.
19. *Kitzur Shulchan Aruch* 32:8.
20. *Treatise on Asthma* 3:6.
21. *Regimen of Health* 1:7.
22. *Medical Aphorisms* 17:34.
23. *Causes of Symptoms* 20.

In general, [the best part of the meat is] the front part and the meat that is attached to the bone, such as the shoulder, chest, ribs.... the intestines, brains, legs and the fats of the abdomen are bad.[24]

FISH

Fish is a food which is easily digested.[25]

The rockfish[26] is tasty, quickly digested and it is suitable for the preservation of health.[27]

Small ocean fish with little fat and white meat that has a pleasant taste, which can be separated easily because it is not sticky, is beneficial since it is digested quickly and has little superfluity. Freshwater fish are not harmful when they come from a large river with clean water.[28]

Large fish that are aged and salted should never be eaten. Large fish should be eaten only in small quantities and only periodically.[29]

24. See *Treatise on Asthma* 3:6.
25. *The Art of Cure* (Rambam), Chapter 7.
26. No further identification.
27. See *Medical Aphorisms* 17:25.
28. *Treatise on Asthma* 3:4; See also *Regimen of Health* 1:9.
29. *Mishneh Torah, Hilchos De'os* 4:9 and 4:10.

IN SUMMARY

Rambam's advice:

- Of the flesh proteins, fish and chicken are the quickest and easiest to digest.

- Choose the lean types of fowl and try to avoid the fatty types.

- Only eat meat if you are bored with chicken.

- Choose the lean types of meat.

- The best parts of the meat are the lean cuts such as those attached to the bone. Avoid the fatty parts such as brains and intestines.

- Try to avoid salty or aged flesh proteins.

- Small fish are usually better than large ones.

APPENDIX D
SHABBOS MEALS
IN HALACHAH

The following excerpts are culled almost verbatim from *Shulchan Aruch* and *Mishnah Berurah*. The sources appear in the footnotes. At the end we will give a summary of the practical implications in halachah.

FOOD AT THE MEALS

There are some authorities who hold that making Shabbos enjoyable (*oneg Shabbos*) is a Torah Law.... Regarding the definition of the mitzvah, the Sages said, "One should make it delightful by eating large fish, heads of garlic." These were distinguished foods in their time. Similarly, one should eat the foods and drinks that are considered delicious in his place according to its custom. Since most people enjoy meat, wine and dainties, it says later that one should eat these foods at the Shabbos meals, according to one's means.[1]

It is good to be careful about having at least two cooked dishes [at each Shabbos meal]. Similarly, it is good to eat fish at each of the three meals, unless fish does not agree with your nature or you dislike fish, because Shabbos was given for enjoyment, not for pain.[2]

1. *Mishnah Berurah* 242:1.
2. Ibid., 242:2.

BREAD AT THE MEALS

The Friday night and Shabbos morning meals cannot be held without bread.[3]

That is, even according to the lenient opinion that one does not have to eat bread at the third Shabbos meal. All authorities agree that the first two meals require bread.[4]

SEUDAH SHELISHIS – THE THIRD SHABBOS MEAL

One should be very careful to eat the third Shabbos meal.[5] Women are obligated to eat the third Shabbos Meal.[6]

One must eat bread at the third Shabbos meal. Some authorities hold that one can eat *mezonos*. Some authorities hold that one can eat meat and fish but not fruit. Other authorities hold that one can eat fruit for this third meal. [7]

According to all views, the most preferred way is with bread and with *lechem mishneh*. The difference of opinion [above] is only whether *bediavad* one has fulfilled his obligation with these other foods.[8]

---

3. *Shulchan Aruch, Orach Chaim* 275:4.
4. *Mishnah Berurah* 275:9.
5. *Mishnah Berurah* 291:1 writes that the source of having three meals is based on an *asmachta* from a verse in the Torah. The reward for eating three meals is also mentioned. The *Aruch HaShulchan* also writes about the importance of eating this third meal.
6. *Shulchan Aruch, Orach Chaim* 291:6.
7. Ibid., 291:5.
8. *Mishnah Berurah* 291:23.

The first opinion, that one should eat bread, is the one to be followed unless one is overly satiated.[9]

Even if one is sated, one can fulfill [the obligation to eat bread at this meal] with a piece of bread the size of a *kebeitzah*, i.e. slightly more than the size of an egg. Some authorities hold that *lechatchilah* a *kezayis* of bread is sufficient. However, it is fitting *lechatchilah* to follow the stringent view if one is able. [10]

If one is unable to eat at all, one is not obligated to cause oneself suffering by eating. But a wise man plans ahead by not filling his stomach at the earlier meal, in order to leave room for the third meal.[11] For otherwise it can result in gross overeating (*achilah gasah*), which is not considered eating.[12]

THE SATURDAY NIGHT MEAL – MELAVEH MALKAH

One should arrange his table after Shabbos in order to escort the Shabbos – even if he only eats an olive's bulk of food.[13]

It is implied from the Talmud that *lechatchilah* one should eat bread at this meal. It is also implied that *lechatchilah* one should eat meat or other cooked foods at this meal. However, if one is afraid of overeating – as, for example, during the summer when the third

---

9. *Shulchan Aruch, Orach Chaim* 291:5.
10. *Mishnah Berurah* 291:2.
11. *Shulchan Aruch, Orach Chaim* 291:1.
12. *Mishnah Berurah* 291:4.
13. *Shulchan Aruch, Orach Chaim* 300:1.

Shabbos meal is eaten close to evening – one should eat *mezonos* or at least fruit.[14]

KIDDUSH WITHOUT A MEAL

The Geonim write that one fulfills the requirement of *kiddush bimkom seudah* by drinking a *revi'is*[15] of wine (alone).[16]

One should not follow this lenient view unless there is a pressing need.[17] (This is regarding Kiddush at night, but one may rely on this view for Kiddush in the day.[18]) Everyone agrees that eating fruit does not fulfill this requirement.

KIDDUSH AND BREAD AMOUNTS

Women are obligated to recite Kiddush.[19]

One must drink the amount of a *melo lugmav* from the Kiddush cup, i.e. the amount which if one will move the liquid to one side of his or her mouth, it will give the appearance that the cheek is full.[20] This amount is determined by one's personal *melo lugmav*, in accordance with one's size. For most people, this amount is the

---

14. *Mishnah Berurah* 300:1.
15. Ibid., 273:22; somewhat more than three fluid ounces (about 86 ml.).
16. *Shulchan Aruch, Orach Chaim* 273:5.
17. *Mishnah Berurah* 273:25.
18. See *Sha'ar HaTziyun* 273:25:29.
19. *Shulchan Aruch, Orach Chaim* 271:2.
20. Ibid., 271:13.

greater part of a *revi'is* measure. One is never required to drink more than a *revi'is*.[21]

The most preferable manner of performing the mitzvah is that the entire group partakes of the Kiddush wine,[22] i.e. a mere taste of wine. Only one of the group is required to drink the amount of *melo lugmav*.[23]

There are those who hold that one who eats less than a *kebeitzah* of bread, washes his hands but does not say the blessing.[24]

One says *birkas ha-mazon* after eating a *kezayis* of bread.[25]

One who eats less than a *kezayis* of bread is not required to wash his hands.[26]

FRUIT BETWEEN MEALS

One should eat numerous fruit...during Shabbos in order to complete the minimum daily requirement to make one hundred blessings.[27] This is because there are fewer blessings in each *Amidah* prayer of Shabbos.[28]

21. *Mishnah Berurah* 271:68.
22. *Shulchan Aruch, Orach Chaim* 271:14.
23. *Mishnah Berurah* 271:71.
24. *Shulchan Aruch, Orach Chaim* 158:2.
25. *Mishnah Berurah* 158:2.
26. *Shulchan Aruch, Orach Chaim* 158:3; See also *Mishnah Berurah* 158:3.
27. *Shulchan Aruch, Orach Chaim* 290:1.
28. *Mishnah Berurah* 290:2.

THE OBLIGATION TO EAT BREAD AT THE MEALS

I asked the following question to three well-known halachic authorities (*poskim*) and received three different opinions:

QUESTION: Regarding eating bread at the meals, all authorities agree that the first two meals require bread. At the third meal, everyone agrees that *lechatchilah* one should eat bread, but there is a difference of opinion whether *bediavad* one has fulfilled his obligation with *mezonos*, meat and fish or fruit. At the Saturday night meal (*melaveh malkah*) we are more lenient, and while it is best to eat bread, if one is afraid of overeating he may eat *mezonos* or at least fruit.

This is said by the *Shulchan Aruch* and *Mishnah Berurah* regarding a regular healthy person. Does this apply to an obese person or to someone who is concerned about their weight?

- One *posek* told me that there is no difference between an obese person and a regular healthy person. One should eat bread at all the meals including *melaveh malkah*. However, one may eat a *kezayis* of bread as explained above.

- Another *posek* told me that one must eat bread at the three Shabbos meals but eating bread at the Saturday night meal is more like a *chumrah*.

- A third *posek* told me that the above laws apply to a regular healthy person, but someone who is obese or someone who is watching their weight and does not eat bread more than once a day during the week, can eat fruit for the third meal and certainly for the Saturday night meal.

As you can see, there are different opinions regarding this subject. Once you familiarize yourself regarding the different possibilities, you should speak to your personal competent halachic authority before implementing any of these more lenient views.

IN SUMMARY

— Some of the earlier authorities hold that making Shabbos enjoyable (*oneg Shabbos*) is a Torah Law. Regarding the definition of this mitzvah, the Sages said that one should eat the foods and drinks that are considered delicious in his place according to its custom.

— Women are obligated the same as men in these laws.

— All authorities agree that the first two meals require bread. Regarding the amount of bread to be eaten, one must eat slightly more than a kebeitzah of bread.

— A *kezayis* is the amount of food that will displace slightly less than one fluid ounce of water (i.e. its volume is 28.8 cubic centimeters). According to the ruling authorities, one may *lechatchilah* eat this amount and make an after blessing.[29] (See Chapter 13 for a table which illustrates the bread amounts of a *kezayis* and a *kebeitzah*.) *Lechatchilah* one should eat a *kezayis* within three minutes. *Bediavad*, four minutes is acceptable.[30]

Continued on next page

29. This is true even according to the Chazon Ish. See *Halachos of K'zayis*, page 20.
30. *Halachos of K'zayis*, page 28.

- On Shabbos, one thin slice of challah the size of a slice of white bread or a quarter of a two-ounce challah roll or a whole machine matzah is more than enough to fulfill the requirement of eating bread at the meals.[31]

- People who feel that this will ruin their diet and detract from enjoying Shabbos can eat just a *kezayis*. However, if you eat this amount of bread you should wash your hands before eating but get someone else to include you in his or her blessing of *al netilas yadayim*.

- For Kiddush, the most preferable manner of performing the mitzvah is that the entire group has a small taste of the Kiddush wine. But as long as the amount of *melo lugmav* is drunk by any one of the group (it does not have to be the person saying Kiddush), no one else is required to drink any wine.

- If a woman wants to make Kiddush on Shabbos morning before the meal but does not want to eat *mezonos*, she can drink a *revi'is* (somewhat more than three fluid ounces) of wine *plus* a *melo lugmav*. She does not have to repeat Kiddush at the meal according to most opinions.

- One must not force himself to eat foods that he dislikes – Shabbos was given to enjoy.

31. See ibid., page 105.

APPENDIX E
INTERNET REFERENCES

INTRODUCTION

1. American Heart Association, "Heart and Stroke Statistics," http://www.heart.org/HEARTORG/General/Heart-and-Stroke-Association-Statistics_UCM_319064_SubHomePage.jsp

CHAPTER 1

1. BBC News, "Chocolate Has Health Benefits," http://news.bbc.co.uk/2/hi/health/4371867.stm

2. CNN, "Chocolate: A Heart-Healthy Confection?" http://faculty.missouri.edu/~glaserr/212woo/group_18_project1.html

3. USA Today, "Study Touts Coffee's Health Benefits," http://www.usatoday.com/news/health/2005-08-28-coffee-antioxidants_x.htm?csp=34

4. BBC NEWS, "Coffee Is 'Health Drink,' Says Italian," http://news.bbc.co.uk/1/hi/world/europe/3540729.stm

5. CNN, "Study Suggests Link between Aspartame and Brain Cancer," http://www.cnn.com/health/9611/18/aspartame/

6. CNN, "Link Between Aspartame, Brain Tumors Dismissed by FDA, Cancer Group," http://www.cnn.com/health/9611/18/nfm/

CHAPTER 4

1. Rand Research Report (May 18, 2006), "The Health Risks of Obesity: Worse Than Smoking, Drinking, or Poverty," http://www.rand.org/pubs/research_briefs/RB4549/index1.html

2. National Institute of Diabetes and Digestive and Kidney Diseases (NIDDK), "Diet and Exercise Dramatically Delay Type 2 Diabetes: Diabetes Medication Metformin Also Effective," http://www.nih.gov/news/pr/aug2001/niddk-08.htm

CHAPTER 6 – PHASE 1, WEEK 1

1. WebMd, *Elaine Magee, MPH, RD*, "6 Foods and Tips for More Fiber," http://www.webmd.com/diet/features/6-foods-and-tips-for-more-fiber

CHAPTER 6 – PHASE 1, WEEK 2

1. See American Council of Exercise, "Before You Start an Exercise Program," http://www.acefitness.org/acefit/healthy_living_fit_facts_content.aspx?itemid=2612

2. See Centers for Disease Control and Prevention, "Why Strength Training?" http://www.cdc.gov/physicalactivity/growingstronger/why

3. The American Heart Association, "Physical Activity," http://www.heart.org/HEARTORG/GettingHealthy/PhysicalActivity/Physical-Activity_UCM_001080_SubHomePage.jsp

4. http://cdc.gov/nccdphp/sgr/prerep.htm

5. Len Kravitz, Ph.D., "Exploring the Mysteries of Exercise," http://www.unm.edu/~lkravitz/Article%20folder/mysteries.html

6. National Institute of Mental Health, "Depression Can Break Your Heart," http://www.chestercountypsychology.com/pdf/DepressionCanBreakYourHeart.pdf

CHAPTER 6 — PHASE 1, WEEK 3

1. "Cancer Trends Progress Report: Fruit and Vegetable Consumption," National Cancer Institute, Division of Cancer Control and Population Sciences, http://progressreport.cancer.gov/doc_detail.asp?pid=1&did =2007&chid=71&coid=707

CHAPTER 6 — PHASE 1, WEEK 4

1. George L. Blackburn, Dietary Patterns for Weight Management and Health," Obesityresearch.Org, http://onlinelibrary.wiley.com/ doi/10.1038/oby.2001.120/full

2. Andrew M. Prentice, *Section I: Obesity, the Major Health Issue of the Twenty-First Century*, "Overeating: The Health Risks," Obesityresearch.Org, http://onlinelibrary.wiley.com/doi/10.1038/oby.2001.124/full

3. Curt Anderson, "IRS Recognizes Obesity as a Disease", http://www. americanobesity.org/irsObesity.htm

4. Patricia Reaney, "Experts Say 'Portion Distortion' Raises Cancer Risk," http://dukeandthedoctor.com/2010/01/experts-say-portion-distortion-raises-cancer-risk

5. Jennifer Warner, "Controlling Portion Size Helps Promote Lasting Weight Loss," Medicinenet.com, http://www.medicinenet.com/script/main/ art.asp?articlekey=55821

6. "Food and Portion Size," American Diabetes Association, http://www. diabetes.org/food-and-fitness/fitness/weight-loss/food-and-portion-size.html

CHAPTER 7 – PHASE 2

1. "Physical Activity for Everyone: Measuring Physical Activity Intensity –
   Target Heart Rate and Estimated Maximum Heart Rate," Centers for
   Disease Control and Prevention and Health Promotion, http://www.cdc.
   gov/physicalactivity/everyone/measuring/index.html

2. "Growing Stronger – Strength Training for Older Adults," *Why Strength
   Training*? Centers for Disease Control and Prevention, http://www.cdc.
   gov/physicalactivity/growingstronger/why/index.html

CHAPTER 8 – PHASE 3

1. "How Much Physical Activity Do You Need?", Centers for Disease Control
   and Prevention, http://www.cdc.gov/physicalactivity/everyone/
   guidelines/index.html

2. "Physical Activity for Everyone: Measuring Physical Activity Intensity:
   What are Some Examples of Activities and Their Intensity Levels?"
   Centers for Disease Control and Prevention, http://www.cdc.gov/
   physicalactivity/everyone/measuring/index.html

CHAPTER 13

1. "How to Understand and Use the Nutrition Facts Label," U.S.
   Food and Drug Administration, http://www.fda.gov/Food/
   IngredientsPackagingLabeling/LabelingNutrition/ucm274593.htm

2. See http://www.foodpyramid.com/mypyramid and http://www.
   choosemyplate.gov/food-groups/vegetables.html

APPENDIX A

1. Centers for Disease Control and Prevention: "Body Mass Index," http://
   www.cdc.gov/healthyweight/assessing/bmi/index.html

2. "Body Mass Index," http://www.nlm.nih.gov/medlineplus/ency/
   article/007196.htm

ABOUT THE AUTHOR

David Zulberg was born in South Africa. He spent six years researching and writing this book. Now in its seventh printing and translated into Hebrew, *The Life-Transforming Diet* has produced dramatic and life-changing results for thousands of people. Zulberg is an ACE®-certified professional and Health Coach. He also has a MS from Columbia University in New York. Life-Transforming Diet Group Leader opportunities are now available – please see www.lifetransformingdiet.com.